S
L

Laura Mitchell, MCSP, DipTP, is well known in British physiotherapy and obstetric circles, particularly in the teaching field.
She also taught Margaret Morris Movement for many years and
gave a weekly programme of exercises for women over a period
of eighteen months for BBC Radio London. Her book *Simple
Relaxation*: the physiological method for easing tension was
published in 1977 and she then did a series about the method
on BBC *Woman's Hour*. She teaches living anatomy at the
London School of Occupational Therapy.

Barbara Dale began her training in dance at the Arts Educational
Trust. She later did a three-year training course specializing in
Movement at Goldsmiths' College, London, followed by a course
in Mensendieck exercises. She gives classes in exercise and Yoga
at her Bodyworkshops in Westbourne Grove and Chiswick,
London.

Simple Movement

THE WHY AND HOW OF EXERCISE

Laura Mitchell
and Barbara Dale

John Murray

First published 1980
by John Murray (Publishers) Ltd
50 Albemarle Street, London w 1 x 4 BD

Printed in Great Britain by
Butler & Tanner Ltd
Frome and London

British Library Cataloguing in Publication Data

Mitchell, Laura
  Simple movement.
  1. Exercise
  2. Physical fitness
  3. Human locomotion
  I. Title   II. Dale, Barbara
  613.7′1   RA781

  ISBN 0–7195–3785–1
  ISBN 0–7195–3786–X Pbk

To all who enjoy all forms of exercise and dancing, and those who teach them, in the hope that it will enhance their understanding and enjoyment.

'There is no machine yet designed, or ever to be designed, that has more excitement or more majesty than the human body.'
A. C. Guyton, *Function of the Human Body*

Contents

Acknowledgements

I wish to thank the following for helpful conversations, views and wise advice in the preparation of this book: Robin Anderson PhD, FPS, Administrator, Scottish Ballet; Jim Arnott TD MA BLitt, Professor (retired) of Drama at Glasgow University; Martha Arnott, Director, Margaret Morris Movement; Audrey Cook, South Western Arts Council, late of Ballet Joos Dance Co.; Jon Paul Cook, Director of Curriculum at the Dell'Arte School of Mime and Comedy, Blue Lake, California, and Lecturer in the Theatre Dept., Humboldt State University, Arcata, California; Lesley Crozier MCSP DipTP, Lecturer in Physiotherapy at Queen's College, Glasgow; June Grieve BSc, Tutor in Anatomy and Physiology at the London School of Occupational Therapy; Jeanne Harper, teacher of Tai-Chi Chuan; Shelia Harrison MCSP, specialist on health of the pelvic floor; Jim Hastie, Ballet Master, Scottish Opera and Administrator, Margaret Morris Movement; Julie McKenna MCSP, Senior Obstetric Physiotherapist at the Royal Free Hospital, London; John Vasey MCSP DipTP, Lecturer in Physiotherapy at Queen's College, Glasgow; Joan Wilder, teacher of Health and Beauty.

LAURA MITCHELL

I wish to thank: all my teachers and pupils, in particular, Joanna Lewis who taught me the original Mensendieck exercises and my yoga teacher Penelope Nield Smith; Laura Mitchell for her wealth of knowledge which she passes on so freely and for her unbounded enthusiasm for the human body, its functions and movements; Colin White for providing me with studios in which to teach Bodywork; lastly my husband and daughter Rebecca and the rest of my family for their patience and encouragement.

BARBARA DALE

Our thanks are also due to the artist Michael Bartlett; the photographers Malcolm Paisley and John Peel; the model for the photographs, Esmé Newton Dunn; the typist, Pamela Munden, and Roger Hudson of John Murray for his expert guidance.

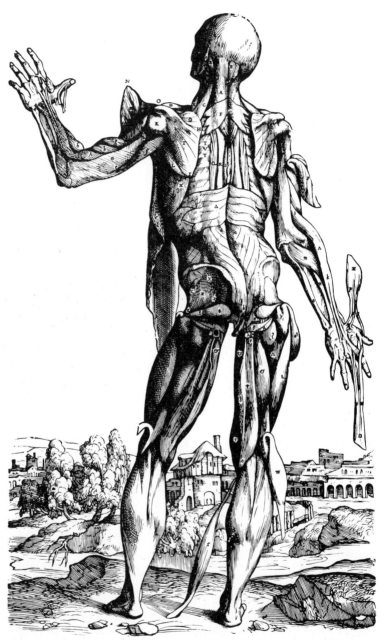

Plate 11 from the second book: *De Humani Corporis Fabrica* by Andreas Vesalius, 1543

1. Giving your body a chance

'I shall examine that true book of ours,
the human body of man himself.'
Vesalius, 1561

This book has been cooking in my brain for many years. I have
wanted to write it for my own interest and in the hope of interesting
others in the structure and function of the human body, and how
it all works together to preserve health, if one gives it a chance.
When, as a physiotherapist, I have been treating patients with exercises to re-educate their muscles, posture or breathing, their interest
has always been stimulated by learning how the appropriate parts
of the body work, and how that affects other parts and functions –
movement of blood, air, abdominal contents, etc. This knowledge,
I am convinced, has helped them to recover faster, and to stay
healthy. Again, when attempting to teach living anatomy to different
types of students, it is obvious that their eyes glaze over at lists of
muscle attachments, but shine with interest when they learn, and
test out for themselves, how muscles, joints, and nerves, work
together in everyday activity. This is what I want the present book
to do; combine theory with practice, anatomy and physiology with
exercises, so that each leavens the other.

Most people hate doing exercises alone. They will cheerfully perform in a class or to music from the radio, if properly encouraged.
But if they are asked whether they have done their exercises they
usually answer that they haven't had time or have forgotten all about
it. And they are quite right. Nothing could be further away from
normal activity than standing alone, trying to find enthusiasm for
performing some apparently meaningless, boring routine that you
have been told by someone else will be 'good for you'. However,
if you understand a little of how this miraculous body of yours
works, and some of the laws which govern it, how things can go
wrong and how you can help the body repair itself, then you are
more likely to look after it better, and enjoy doing so. It is of vital
importance to the quality of your life.

Don't become a sitting duck

Of course if we could lead absolutely natural lives walking, running, hammering, sawing, lifting, throwing – all day long, our joints would be so strong and lubricated, our muscles so developed and accustomed to work, our hearts and breathing apparatus so resilient, that they would respond, and might be trained to any new well-chosen task that we might give them. But most people do not do these movements daily. We sit in car, bus or train to go to work; we often sit at work; we often lean forward continuously while working. We sometimes sit for long periods hunched in a chair, or lie habitually on a soft swaying bed, curled into a ball.

Just take a look at your dog or cat. All that stretching and dashing about is how they keep fit in between bouts of sleeping. Do you keep the oil in your joints moving? Do you stretch freely after you have been fixed in one position for some time, whether at work or watching television?[1] Or do you just sit there getting stiffer and stiffer, with your muscles becoming weak and distorted, your blood circulation, breathing and digestion slowed down, and feeling continuously fatigued? When did you last examine your own work patterns?[2] Are they doing you harm or good?

Distortion and deformity

For many of us work consists in shifting a knob, lifting a telephone, talking, pushing a pencil, pressing cash register buttons, or other slight activity. We have mostly become brain workers, not body workers, and so our muscles become small and weak from lack of use. We may even change our shape, and become actually deformed by some muscles getting tighter, while others become too slack. This can be such a gradual process that one is not aware of it happening over months or even years. For example, I had pain in my hip region for some years which was accentuated when I stood up. So, as well as using a stick in the opposite hand, I also unconsciously developed the habit, when standing, of bending the hip and knee on the bad side, lifting my heel and only resting the front part of my foot on the ground. I put most of my weight on the other leg. Eventually I became aware that I was becoming crooked, and I had to take myself in hand and consciously adopt the correct posture.

This is a typical example of how the body will adapt movements to prevent pain, and how distortion can so easily arise without the person concerned being aware of what is happening. Deformity can increase and cause other trouble in bones, ligaments, muscles and supporting fibrous areas. It can progress, if not prevented, until the person concerned becomes an invalid.

Conforming to the body's laws

We must also remember that we live in a world ruled by the law of gravity, whereby everything is being pulled by its own weight towards the earth all the time. Malformation can arise if effort is not properly directed to overcome the trouble that this pull of gravity can cause. Forward-poking heads, rounded shoulders, arms falling forward, sunken chests, sway backs – all these common defects are often unrecognized by the person concerned, and will lead to further trouble if not corrected.

I have had to treat so many patients who have damaged themselves by doing movements which flouted fundamental laws of the body: double leg raising by women with weak pelvic or abdominal muscles, or head stands by Yoga enthusiasts before they were trained for such abnormal feats. At the beginning of the Second World War, we treated rows of men and women in hospital beds, injured, not by enemy action but by unaccustomed and unsuitable activity. Muscles must work according to their own capabilities and obey mechanical laws. One frequent injury was hernia (rupture), from lifting weights with no knowledge of the correct mechanics of lifting, when the person already had weak abdominal muscles. Another was back injury due to sitting in a cramped, bent-up position, driving a tank over rough ground, when the soldier already had a weak back, not having used it enough when he was a civilian.

Equally it is not safe to 'take up exercise' without careful selection, planning and safeguards. For instance, doctors have recently seen an outburst of joggers' ailments, affecting men and women: bruised feet and nipples, and sometimes joint and muscle strains. These conditions are due to unaccustomed extra friction on these parts, without proper preparation or protection. There have also been other more serious disabilities arising out of too strenuous jogging, without suitable care for the individual involved, and adequate gradual building up of the activity for that person.[3]

Do try to see if you can stop your lifestyle or pattern of work turning your body – the only one of which you are in complete charge – into a well-nigh motionless mass. Equally if you feel some deformity creeping up on you, fight back, really tuning in to your feelings of your joints, fibrous tissue and skin, and appreciate what is happening there. Do not attempt to feel muscles because your conscious brain cannot do this.[4] If you have even a small change in posture or balance, if you have weak muscles, stiff joints, or pain, then you are in danger of developing 'secondary deformities' which may eventually affect every part of you, from faulty circulation of blood to gross crippling. If at all possible, take the trouble to prevent this 'lest a worse fate befall you'.

It would be a great help if schools would emphasize health education more, explaining to children how important exercise is to keep their bodies in good working order, and encourage children in various forms of exercise for its own sake as something for each individual to enjoy, rather than the constant emphasis on competitive sports, as is so often the case in schools today. In this way exercise could be established as an enjoyable habit for life, not something you stop when you stop competing in sporting events later in life.

You have one great asset, one warning bell to which you must always pay attention: pain. Two hundred years ago Voltaire said 'Pain is a vigilant guard against all our dangers, pain loudly tells us over and over again: "Take care, save your life".'[5] The body will tolerate an outrageous amount of abuse and neglect but of course the better we treat it, and understand it, the more it responds in health and a general feeling of well-being. Perhaps this is the moment to remind you that in 1974 the National Health Service bill for tranquillizers was £8,144,000 and in 1977 it was £15·5 million. Even allowing for inflation, that is a hefty increase. Over fifteen *million* pounds spent just to soothe us down! Of course tranquillizers are a necessary help in some conditions, but so many people have told me that they have been able to stop taking them completely, by learning how to relax and by improving their general health by exercise, that I believe this is often possible.

Why another book?

Nowadays fitness is becoming a generally accepted principle of life, whereas thirty to forty years ago it was mainly the domain of the professional athlete, or dancer, and the odd health fanatic. There are numerous teachers of all kinds; some members of accepted professional bodies, and others just purveying their own concoctions, holding classes and telling others what to do. It seems that anybody with a short training, or vague interest in exercise, feels fitted to conduct classes and give advice to the eager. One can hardly open a newspaper without seeing lists of do's and don'ts for fitness and pictures with accompanying descriptions. New books come out every year. So why are we adding yet one more?

Because we think we can offer a measure of knowledge and expertise. We expect the other people who interfere with our bodies, like doctors and dentists, to be highly qualified. Should we not expect as much when we are dealing with overall bodily activity?

I was trained as a physiotherapist in the days when 'medical gymnastics' formed a large part of the training. I later trained in the Margaret Morris Movement in dancing for five years and became the head of the medical side of the training school in London. In 1942 I qualified as a teacher of modern physiotherapy and have been teaching applied anatomy and physiology ever since; firstly full-time to physiotherapy students, and then, when I took up private practice, part-time to occupational therapy students. This I still do. In private practice I specialized in rehabilitation, e.g. orthopaedic and obstetric patients. This led me to the need for a scientific method of relaxation and this I gradually evolved, calling it Physiological Relaxation. In 1963 I was asked to demonstrate this technique at the World Confederation of Physical Therapy in Copenhagen; in 1977 I published a book, *Simple Relaxation: the Physiological Method for Easing Tension*, and in 1978 I broadcast a series on BBC radio *Woman's Hour*. This method is now taught, to my knowledge, in twenty-five countries. It is based upon the fundamental laws which govern all body movements.

I have enlisted the aid of Barbara Dale who has written Chapters 5 and 6. She has chosen to describe a system of exercises based on the Mensendieck method as it is a very explicit one, training movements by the main muscle groups of the body in a pleasant, easily adjusted sequence. We hope that this, as well as giving you exercise, will provide firm points of reference for any more complex and demanding activity which you might later select for yourself.

Barbara Dale writes of herself: 'My training began at a theatrical school where we were taught every kind of dance from Greek to Martha Graham's contemporary style. We took many exams in the different styles and did regular performances. Somehow, I always found myself more involved with leading warming-up and conditioning sessions and helping my friends with their performances, rather than performing myself. Later I found myself in the West Indies and Africa where again I was constantly asked to teach conditioning classes for performers and to give keep-fit classes for non-dancers. I began to devise my own exercise method, combining the conditioning exercises that I had learnt at dance school and the Yoga I have practised since. I also taught this combination when I returned to England. Later I did a course in Mensendieck exercises in London and went on to do the teachers' course. I found the Mensendieck method was a marvellous jumping-off point for people who had not exercised for many years, and who were rather nervous and shy about the whole idea of exercise. I saw too what a tremendous help this gentle form of exercise could be in helping to control migraine headaches, back aches, sore feet and many other aches and pains that afflict so many of us. And so I began to base a great deal of my work on the Mensendieck exercises I had learned.

'During my travels I was also constantly involved in teaching children various kinds of dance classes. I wanted to keep up this side of my work on returning to London but found that no number of dance certificates were enough to win me a place teaching dance in London schools. The answer to my enquiries was always the same – "We do not accept teachers without a general teachers' certificate; dance teachers' certificates are not enough." So, I did a three-year teacher training course specializing in Movement at the University of London's Goldsmiths College. However, after a break to have a child, I find now that my time is taken up with my particular interest of teaching exercise to adults.

'Through the years I have become profoundly interested in helping people to feel better in their everyday lives through improved posture, exercise and relaxation. This is now my main interest and work.'

We see this book as an introductory primer aiming to provide a good foundation for any other system, sport, or pastime anyone cares to add; for instance, Yoga, keep-fit, or modern dancing. Thus, this book in no way seeks to oust the many other excellent systems and accompanying books. It is a companion not a rival: the more exercise classes of different kinds to suit different tastes, the better. The demand is great.

You will find here physiological and anatomical facts and fundamental physical laws – such as gravity and leverage – that affect bodily movement. I have used everyday language throughout. It is my experience that the general public are interested in all this, and if one cuts out jargon and manages to explain clearly what one is trying to say, they are quite capable of understanding. I believe firmly that the more we know of the reasons for, and results of, particular exercises, the better we do them, the more we enjoy doing them, and the less risk there is of us damaging ourselves by doing them wrongly, or indeed, choosing the wrong ones.

In considering the physiological working of the body I shall be trying to explain, in so far as I am able, the normal working of the parts that control and assist movement and also what results we can expect from movement. Of course we all decide for ourselves, whether we want to use the body in a normal way or in some other. For example I shall explain the movements, and their effects, of the chest, and lungs, in what is called 'normal' breathing. In some forms of Yoga training many other kinds of breathing controls are taught. The use of the toes in ballet dancing, as the base for the body, is quite abnormal, but traditional for grace and elegance. Obviously I am not going to mount a campaign against either. This amazing body of ours is so resilient, that it will accommodate all kinds of variations. But surely it is immensely important to understand and appreciate the normal first of all, so that if one wants to deviate from it, at least one is aware of what is happening. Truth is never wasted.

I hope you will find here all the help, encouragement and range of choice you may need to deal with your own selection of exercise. It is always exciting to find you can take more control of your own body – and therefore of your life.

2. Gravity and levers, muscles and nerves

'The design is perfect, physiology
reeks with purpose and design.'
John Stewart Collis[1]

We are apt to imagine that the study of human movement, known
as kinesiology, and the re-education of muscle are modern sciences,
but this is not so. Aristotle, Leonardo da Vinci, Michelangelo and
Vesalius are only a few of those throughout the centuries who were
deeply interested in this aspect of the human body.[2] But in recent
years knowledge of living human movement has advanced on many
fronts. Specialists of all kinds, from anatomists, physiologists,
engineers and mathematicians, to biologists, physicists and psycho-
logists have added their quota and professionalism, so that the amateur, and indeed the teacher, has more and more knowledge to draw
upon.[3] We are in good company when we take the matter seriously,
probe about to get at the scientific foundations of movement, and
are not just content with vague notions of what might be useful or
'good for us'. So let us try to utilize this great flood of learning. Even
if some of the specialized information is beyond our complete com-
prehension, it is good to realize how much research has been and
is being done.

Gravity

The human body is ruled by those physical laws that affect everything in the world. For example the earth exerts attraction on everything within its gravitational field, i.e. pull, and thus produces what
we feel as weight. If you put your hand under the tummy of a kitten
and lift it up, you will find you can do so very easily, but if you
put your hand under the tummy of a large cat you might not be
able to lift it at all. You would say it was too heavy; in other words,
it was attracted to the earth perhaps ten times more than the kitten.
And even this attraction is not constant. If you took the cat to the
North or South Pole it would weigh heavier, and if you took it to
the Equator, it would weigh less.[4] We are even told by botanists
that it is gravity that helps the roots of plants grow into the earth.

It is generally accepted that we don't quite understand the nature of gravity, but like many laws of the universe we may not fully understand, it still works and influences us all.

People are not surprised when they stand on the scales and it registers their weight as so many pounds, yet when I tell them their head weighs about 12 lbs (5 kg) they are often amazed. Normally authorities list the parts as a percentage of the whole body weight. But this is difficult to grasp. Here is a list of the approximate weights of all your various parts, assuming you weighed 150 lbs. [5]

2 Feet	3 lbs each	=	6 lbs
2 Lower legs	7 ,, ,,	=	14 ,,
2 Thighs	15 ,, ,,	=	30 ,,
1 Trunk	70 ,, ,,	=	70 ,,
2 Upper arms	5 ,, ,,	=	10 ,,
2 Forearms	4 ,, ,,	=	8 ,,
2 Hands	1 ,, ,,	=	2 ,,
1 Head	10 ,, ,,	=	10 ,,
			150 lbs

Of course all weights of parts vary with the individual; we have only to look at a crowd of people to be sure of this. Here is a table of weight distribution done on the basis of materials rather than finished structure, for a man weighing 154 lbs (70 kg). [6]

ORGANS OR TISSUES	PERCENTAGE OF BODY WEIGHT
Muscles	43
Fat	14
Bone and marrow	14
Viscera	12
Connective tissue and skin	9
Blood	8
	100

One must remember that all figures are variable and that 65 per cent of adult body weight is water. You may be amused to hear that the adult brain, of which we are apt to be so proud, is about 2 per cent of body weight.

R. D. Lockhart in his book *Living Anatomy*[7] suggests the following differences between men and women. Men's muscles are 42 per cent of body weight and their fat is 18 per cent of body weight. Women's muscles are 36 per cent of body weight and their fat is 28 per cent of body weight. This is important to realize. I have sometimes found that some women, who are imbued with the idea of male and female equality, forget little fundamental details like this.[8] But facts are facts – so when your boy friend offers to carry the heavy suitcase he is being sensible, and you are only being silly if you don't let him. His muscles are naturally bigger and stronger – *vive la différence*. Also the female body is naturally rounded by the extra little layer of fat. Beware of too drastic slimming.

All parts of you are being pulled towards the earth by the force of gravity registered as their own weight all day long. So no wonder you get tired and want 'to take the weight off your feet'. Given the sedentary lives we lead, exercise is not only the concern of the sportsman or the slimmer these days; you need to exercise just to keep your muscles able to do the job of lifting bits of yourself, and indeed your whole weight, from place to place. Alan Moorehead in his book *The White Nile*[9] tells of Bugandan women so fat, because their men so preferred them, that they had to be rolled from place to place. At least most of us have not reached that stage yet.

If you are a typist and lean the ten or twelve pounds of your head forward all day long, it has to be supported and held by the muscles at the back of your neck, just as a little boy holds a fishing rod with a fish at the end of the line. If he let go, the fish would fall. If the muscles at the back of your neck are not in good health and strength and able to work well, they, too, want to let go the weight. If you continue to make them work so inconveniently, they become strained, uncomfortable, and sodden with their own waste products, through lack of proper blood flow (see p. 42). Eventually some area will give way, and result in headaches or displaced discs, or worn neck joints, or fibrositis (which is inflammation of the fibrous parts of muscle), or localized muscle spasm, swelling, etc. All these conditions are frequently found. Pain will sooner or later scream at you that all is not well.

Relentless gravity was pulling your head more than the supporting muscles could comfortably control. So, since you can't change the gravitational pull (i.e. the weight of your head) you have to strengthen the muscles doing the job and deal with any other changes that may have resulted, e.g. poor blood supply, squashed joints, etc. (See chap. 5 for safe neck exercises).

CENTRE OF GRAVITY

This example leads us to pay some attention to the centre of gravity of anything – ourselves, parts of ourselves, or anything else. The centre of gravity of an object is the point of balance, that means the imaginary point about which all the surrounding masses are equal. In the body this is considered to be towards the upper part of the back of the pelvis (second sacral) when standing, but of course it will vary with the shape of the person. Anyone with a very heavy top half or carrying a heavy object in their arms would cause their centre of gravity to become higher in order to get the weight above and below the point equal. Any weight added to the lower half will bring the centre of gravity lower. The nearer the centre of gravity gets to the base, the more stable an object is.

The base is that part of any object that is on the ground. In the standing human being it is the part of the ground on which the two feet rest and the part of the ground between. In sitting it is the area enclosed by the legs of the chair plus the area of the feet. The line of gravity is a vertical line from the ground which passes through the centre of gravity. The more central the position of this line within the base, the more stable is the object. The more it nears the edge of the base, the more unstable and, if it goes outside the base, the object falls over. In the human being muscles start working immediately this danger threatens so as to prevent this (see chap. 4), and thus we regain our balance.

Small children have a high centre of gravity as their top half is much heavier than their lower half, since the muscles of the legs are relatively undeveloped till they walk and run.[10] How often has one watched the tottering gait of the toddler as he swayed around and finally fell. He was trying to cope with his line of gravity falling outside the small base of his little foot as he transferred his weight from one to the other, and with his high centre of gravity this was very difficult. But up he got again for another try, and thus he developed his muscles for balancing, and his balance control system.

All balance exercises, dancing and sports, are of value in maintaining this muscular power and control. The smaller the base the greater the muscular power and co-ordination needed to keep the line of gravity within it. Think of the control of a ballet dancer performing a pirouette on point, or an acrobat balancing on one hand for an instant as he turns cartwheels. Think of the beauty of a woman carrying a water pot on her head: she looks delightful because her body has not become distorted in any way. The extra weight has been added at the top of her line of gravity and, as it were, become part of her. She has developed her muscular skill to cope with the raised centre of gravity.

When we carry a heavy suitcase in one hand, we have to compensate for the extra weight at one side by bending to the other side, or sometimes by raising the opposite arm, to maintain balance. If our work, whether it be lifting bundles in a shop or our own children at home, demands that we do this often, we will be forcing our muscles to work in a very tiring way. Due thought should be given to any repetitive action as to whether it is being happily and healthily coped with by the working muscles or whether these are liable to break down under the strain and further damage result. The law of gravity is inexorable.

Levers

If you are only vaguely interested in exercise you may find what follows a bit complicated, but I hope you will read on, because it is essential to understand a little of the laws which govern you, if you want to get full benefit from Chapters 5 and 6. I must also include some basic information for teachers, and for those who are going to perform professionally, e.g. ballet students.

The other physical law governing all muscle work, as well as gravity, is the law of leverage[11] which, although you are probably quite unaware of it, you use all day long. Everyone, I am sure, has applied this law to get the top off a tin which has become stuck. You push some strong piece of metal like a coin, under the stiff lid, and, as we say 'lever it up'. Suppose it comes up immediately, that means the power you exerted downwards was greater than the gravitational pull (weight) of the stuck lid. Now, suppose the lid didn't come up or the metal you were using bent or slipped, you would immediately look for a longer, stronger piece of metal, a safer 'fulcrum', i.e. resting place, and then applying it as before, you could lift the lid.

As Archimedes, the Greek scientist who discovered the principle of leverage, said, 'Give me but one firm spot on which to stand, and I will move the earth.'[12] The other requirement apart from the firm spot, in the operation of this law, is that you must have a rigid bar of some kind, and power or force applied to that bar. You can then lift weight with it.

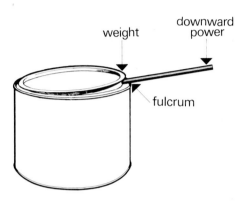

We have all seen this principle applied to a see-saw. Tiny little Toby can lift big fat brother, on the other end. Why? Because he has applied Archimedes' principle. The 'firm spot' is the fulcrum on which the see-saw rests and about which it can move. The rigid bar is the see-saw. Toby is the power or force and his big brother is the weight registered through his line of gravity. Now the reason he can lift big brother is because he has a longer bit of the see-saw on his side of the fulcrum than big brother has on his side. This length multiplied by Toby's weight will be greater than big brother's weight multiplied by his short piece of see-saw.

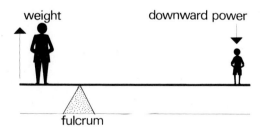

And so we have arrived at the laws of leverage. The Power Arm is that bit of the rigid bar from the fulcrum to the point where power is applied (Toby). The Weight Arm is that bit of the rigid bar from the fulcrum to the point where weight is registered (big brother). The formula is Power Arm × Power = Weight Arm × Weight.

In the body exactly the same principle is applied in pulling the head backwards (extending).

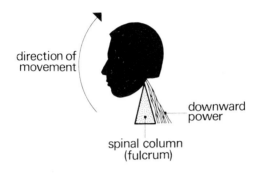

direction of movement

downward power

spinal column (fulcrum)

This is called a first-class lever because the fulcrum is always some-where between the weight, in this case, the head, and the power. The great advantage, therefore, is that it is very stable. The previous example of the see-saw was also a first-class lever.

Of course in the body the rigid bar is not always a convenient rigid bit of bone like the skull. It is an arm, leg, foot, or the trunk, and often it is made shorter or longer by bending up a limb, or straightening it out. Convenient muscles will work to maintain the rigidity, for example over the elbow or knee joint. This is true also of the trunk or foot, when they are supposed to be acting as rigid bars held firmly by muscles. If these muscles give way the rigid bar collapses, and so we have a damaged spine or foot. It is to help to prevent this kind of accident that we are bothering with all this. We saw in the stuck lid experiment that the rigid bar might bend or the fulcrum slip if the weight or the power applied was greater than they could bear. And so it is in the human body.

In the arm and leg the leverage arrangement is different from that in the neck. Let us consider drinking a cup of coffee. This time the fulcrum is the elbow joint because that is where the rigid bar, which is the lower arm, is tied on by ligaments but in such a way as to allow it to move. The fulcrum is therefore found to be at one end while the weight is at the other end. The weight is not merely the cup of coffee but the forearm and hand as well. The power is obviously the flexor muscles of the elbow because they are pulling up the forearm so that you can put the coffee cup to your mouth. Notice, it is not the position of the main bulk of the working muscles which matters, but the point at which their tendons attach to the lever. The power of the working muscles is being exerted where they attach to the bones of the forearm. This is just below the elbow onto both bones (biceps into radius, and brachialis into ulna). The power is therefore applied between the fulcrum and the weight. If we want to relate this movement to the law of leverage, then the power arm is the bit of the forearm between the elbow and the point where the working muscles attach to the forearm, and the weight arm is the *whole* forearm from elbow to cup.

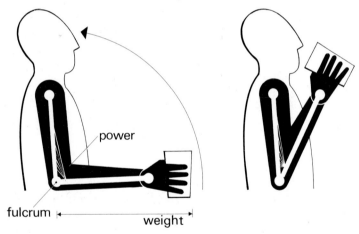

This arrangement is called a third-class lever and most work in the body is carried out in this way. It is a good bargain. Every time we eat or drink, our hand reaches our mouth with only a small movement at the elbow joint and a relatively small muscle shortening. Because we are using a third-class lever we shift the weight a much larger distance than the movement in the joint involved.[13]

The same performance takes place with shoulder movements when we move things in our hands and even more so if we attach added length of lever by holding a stick, racquet or fishing rod.[14]

Doob ~~Doobey~~ Bros

Minute By Minute ~ LP

"What A Fool Believes".

Just think of the distance an experienced fisherman can throw the fly with only a small movement of his shoulder joint. The Aborigines use a throwing stick in which they have a hole which houses the end of their spear. They can then throw the spear a much greater distance than would have been possible with the spear in the hand, because they have lengthened the lever. Moving down the body, when you kick with a straight leg, the foot describes a much larger part of a circle than the top of the leg bone (femur) at the hip joint.

The leverage principle can also be applied with the fulcrum at one end, the power at the other end, and the weight between them. This is a second-class lever and kinesiologists are divided as to whether any are found in the body. Some say they are used in raising the body on the toes or pulling the jaw down.[15]

Applying the laws of gravity and leverage

Suppose you have weak or damaged muscles or joints that you are trying to make strong. If you give them heavy work, too early, they will not respond by strengthening, but instead something will be damaged, as in the beginning of the lid experiment. You cannot change the placing of the joint and muscle attachments; the only thing you can change in training is the weight arm, by making it longer or shorter, and/or by adding or taking away weight. If you bend up the arm at the elbow so that the fingers rest on the shoulder you have literally halved the length, and this is the same as reducing the weight, because the law is

$$\text{Power} \times \text{power arm} = \text{Weight} \times \text{weight arm}$$

By exercising in this position the weak muscles all round the shoulder can be strengthened gradually. When this is achieved you then perform the same movements with the whole arm stretched out, thus increasing the work to be done, by increasing the length of the weight arm. This is easy to do in the body: you simply hold intermediate joints firm with other muscles.

Finally you can hold carefully graduated weights in the hand to increase the work still more; or if more convenient, add length by holding a cane, racquet, or hockey stick; or both length and weight can be increased.

As the muscles gain power you can safely increase their capacity for work from A→B→C→D→E. If, however, you had begun at E

A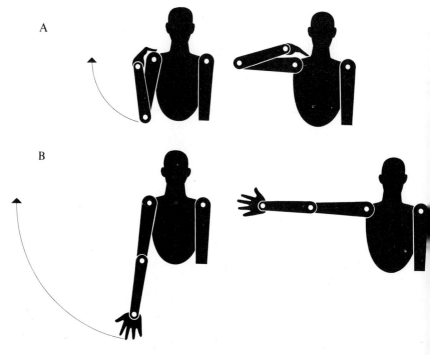

B

Five variations on one exercise, gradually increasing muscle work by applying the laws of leverage

A   exercise halving the length of the weight arm
B   the same exercise as A, but with the weight arm lengthened
C   with added weight
D   with added length
E   with added length and weight

C

D

E

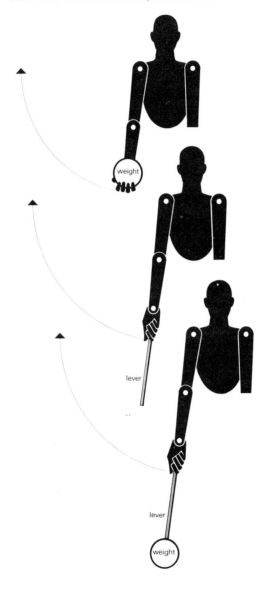

you might have damaged the tendons, or muscles, or joint, and so caused harm instead of the increased muscle power and efficiency you had hoped for. Every day hundreds of people damage themselves by doing just this. If someone lifts a weight – perhaps one of his children – and swings him around, he will be using a third-class lever with added weight *and* length at the end of the weight arm. This then becomes a formidable task and unless the joints of his arms and spine are stable enough, and the muscles of his arms and back strong enough to sustain it, either the muscles or some joints will give way and be damaged. Instead of a child the object might be a heavy axe suddenly used by a week-end gardener, or a large suitcase being swung into the boot of a car. These are common causes of damage to muscles or discs or joints of the spinal column.

If the arm and trunk muscles are gradually strengthened and the shoulder and spinal joints kept mobile by simple movements, then we can attempt to handle all kinds of heavy objects with ease and safety. The same principles of training can be applied to each segment of the body.

All activities involving balance make body muscles work. Just standing on one leg can be a difficult and useful exercise for some people, due to the smallness of the base and the constant adjustments required to keep the line of gravity within the base. Performing exercises or dance movements with the hands above the head increases the muscle work and co-ordination because of the rise in the centre of gravity. Work can be gradually increased by standing with feet apart to begin with, then together, then on one foot, then rising on the toes. Control of momentum can be added by moving the whole body on the toes in various directions. Children enjoy balancing, so climbing trees, ladders, frames and onto each other, as in pyramid building, are all very useful forms of training.

Nowadays, since the laws of gravity and leverage have come to be so much appreciated in training muscles, all kinds of devices are used to diminish or increase the effect of gravity, i.e. weight, and length of lever.

Weightless exercises are an excellent way of reducing muscle work. Of course there is no such thing as a completely weightless movement. There is always some friction, water resistance, or air pressure, but it is a useful term. It means the weight of the moving part has been transferred to something else as in swimming, or exercises in suspension, or by pulleys. Gradually weight can be increased. Weight or lever length can be added in all sorts of ways: holding balls, hoops, scarves, flags of various sizes on flag poles of graduated length etc. All these, children love using. For adults, spring resistance, measured and increasing weights and levers are recommended.[16] All forms of dancing, sports, and ball games call for control of weight, leverage, and momentum.[17]

Muscle

Muscle can do extraordinary things: change its shape, get bigger, smaller, pull bones about, open up spaces, close spaces – like opening and shutting your mouth – and even move your whole body at any pace you choose. Various groups of muscles work together in different ways to meet some particular demand that you may make. If you decide to drive a large nail into a tough piece of wood with a big hammer, you unconsciously get a quite different muscle programme activity from your nervous system for the performance, than if you wish to use a tiny hammer for hammering jewellery. You also get a change of heart beat, blood pressure, diversity of blood circulation and type of breathing as you continue with each operation. So when we are studying muscle we are investigating other systems of the body at the same time. They all work together.

There are three types of muscle in the body – cardiac in the heart, involuntary in blood vessels, stomach and intestines, and voluntary attached to bones. The last is the one which particularly concerns us here, and we can leave the other two types. Voluntary is so called from the Latin word *voluntas* meaning 'will', because the action of these muscles is under the control of the will. Voluntary muscle is made up of fibres in varying formations to promote strength or exactness of performance. There may be hundreds in small muscles or thousands in large muscles. To function muscle must have sufficient blood circulation and an intact nerve containing hundreds of fibres. One nerve fibre may control anything from one muscle fibre, as in the eye, to hundreds of fibres, depending on the function of the muscles concerned; the small muscles of the thumb have far fewer muscle fibres per nerve fibre than the gross muscles moving the hip joint. So we can expect minute movements in the eye, exact movements from the thumb such as directing a pencil, threading a needle,

etc. and only very large movements at the hip joint. The diagram
below shows the amounts of the motor area of the conscious brain
devoted to different parts of the body. The lips and the hands have
by far the greatest areas. The trunk has rather less than the toes,
while the whole long legs have less than the arms and hands. We
should use this knowledge when trying to direct our own or other
people's exercises.

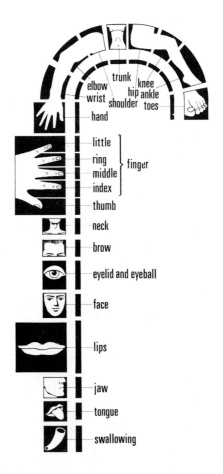

Movement control in the brain. The amounts of the motor area of the conscious brain devoted to different parts of the body

Muscle fibres are only about 1 cm to 4 cms in length, bound together in bundles. Fibrous tissue covers the bundles and lies between them, and eventually joins together to form the tendon which usually inserts into bone to lever it about.[18] Some muscles do not insert into bone but into fibrous tissues, e.g. the mouth, or midline of the abdomen, or pelvic floor (see chap. 3 p. 54). The result of contraction of muscle is determined by the direction of the muscle fibres, and the placing of its attachments into fibrous tissue or bone. The shape of the joints involved also rules what movement is possible. In ball and socket joints, like the hip and shoulder, movement in all directions is possible, but in hinge joints like the elbow and fingers, only movement in two directions (flexion and extension) can be produced by the muscles. No other movement should be attempted by forcible manipulation or harm may be done.

Smaller body segments can move faster than larger ones. Here is an interesting comparative list of wing beats which illustrates this.[19]

Humming bird	200 per second	
Sparrow	13 ,,	,,
Pigeon	8 ,,	,,
Stork	2 ,,	,,

Contractions of mouth muscles in eating also decrease as the mouth gets bigger:

White mouse	350 per minute	
Human	90–100 per minute	
Ox	70 ,,	,,

Therefore you would expect to be able to perform quicker movements with your fingers or hands, than with your whole arm or whole leg. You are also able to perform different kinds of exercise using the same joints because you have various types of muscles surrounding each joint.

FUNCTION OF MUSCLE

Look in a mirror and tell your mouth to make as small a circle as possible. Now tell it to remain small. Now tell your mouth to become as wide a circle as possible. Again you will see it do so immediately. Now tell it to remain large and then to STOP. It will perform all this easily, and when you say stop it will return to its original shape. Now tell your nose to become smaller and then bigger. Of course it won't. Your mouth is mainly composed of muscle but your nose is just a blob of fibrous tissue and fat, with a few short muscles at either side to twitch it about.

As you moved your mouth you have proved to yourself the functions of muscle which are unique –

1. It can carry out instructions for a finished performance, although you are not aware exactly how you do this.
2. It can become smaller and return to its original shape.
3. It can be stretched and return to its original shape.
4. It can work both when it is getting smaller and also when it has been stretched.
5. It can hold a chosen position.
6. It can stop all activity, i.e. relax.[20]

Muscles occasionally work separately but usually do so in groups for a purpose: moving bones, stabilizing joints, or pulling on fibrous tissue. As you have just proved, muscles have special jobs that they will perform. Some muscles have more than one action: the biceps first turns over the forearm (supination) so that the palm of the hand is directed upwards and will then help to bend up (flex) the elbow with the rest of the group of elbow flexors.

TYPES OF MUSCLE WORK

Nerve impulses pass along nerves in rapid succession, frequently at speeds up to 100 metres per second (about the distance of a football field). When they are received by the muscular tissue they cause a chemical change; this causes an electrical change and then an electrical current to flow. This in turn causes the muscle material to change in shape, that is, to contract. This is muscle work.[21]

Muscles work in three ways:[22]

1. Concentric (Isotonic). They work and shorten.
2. Eccentric (Isotonic). They work as they are gradually stretched by the weight of the part (gravity) or something else, e.g. a spring, but they control the rate of movement.
3. Static (Isometric). They work and remain the same length.

Take as an example, the muscles at your shoulder joint.

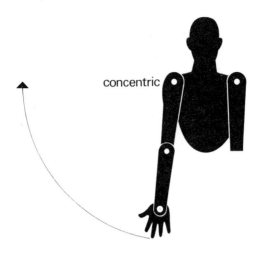

Concentric. Muscles (abductors of shoulder joint) shorten to take arm up sideways to shoulder level.

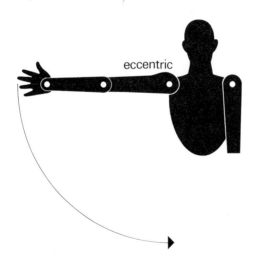

Eccentric. The same muscles work to control the rate at which the arm is lowered, against the pull of gravity. If they did not work, the arm would just fall down.

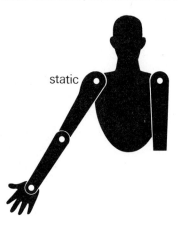

Static. The same muscles work, but without getting shorter or longer, to hold the arm in a selected position against gravity.[23]

In all three instances the opposing muscles (adductors of shoulder joint) are completely relaxed.[24]

Eccentric muscle work is the easiest to perform. It is most used in the body to control the weight of our limbs against the pull of gravity. Concentric is next, then static, which is the most tiring. The number of fibres working is decided by the work to be done: the more work either by weight or leverage, the more fibres working. Each fibre works fully or not at all; this is the All or None Law. We now know by experiment, that if a muscle is not given any work to do, it relaxes completely. We used to think it always remained in slight contraction (see Ref. 20). The bulk of each muscle depends upon the individual's personal physique and also upon use. Use develops the size of muscle fibres, although there is no increase in the number of fibres. Working against resistance makes muscles stronger, static muscle work especially builds bulk. Short sharp bursts of varied activity with suitable rests are preferable to longer sessions of gentle performance.

COLOUR OF MUSCLE

Some muscles are capable of strong movements and of sustaining a part of the body in a particular posture, other muscles are particularly designed for quick activity. Thus we use the deep muscle of the calf (soleus) when standing, as it is attached above to the bones of the lower leg and below onto the heel by the Achilles tendon, while we use the muscle which forms the curved bulk of the calf (gastrocnemius) to perform strong, quick movements as in jumping and dancing. It is attached above the knee onto the femur, and at its lower end also into the heel by the Achilles tendon. The soleus has closely packed bundles of fibres, more blood cells and is therefore dark reddish in colour whereas the gastrocnemius, although larger, is finer in texture and whiter. These correspond to the dark and white meat in a chicken. My wise old Siamese cat would only eat dark meat so there must be a vast difference in substance. In exercising the muscles around the ankle one should be sure to include both slow, sustained, and quick activity.

MUSCLE RANGES

What is called the full range of a muscle is from its most stretched point to its most contracted. The outer range is from the most stretched to midpoint, and the inner range from midpoint to its most contracted. A muscle works best after it has been stretched[25] but not overstretched. This weakens muscle. It is therefore at its most efficient if it can be fully stretched and then fully contracted, its most powerful moment being at midpoint in this excursion.

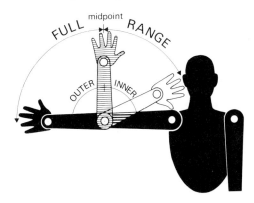

Inner range work is most satisfactory and has a helpful squeezing action on the local circulation. It squeezes out capillary blood forward towards the veins and thus helps to get rid of waste products (see p. 42). It is thus not tiring and can continue happily for some time. Conveying food to the mouth is inner range muscle work for the flexors of the elbow, and we find this quite pleasant work.

Outer range work is the most tiring, and if the muscle work is also static, it is very tiring indeed (see p. 36). We are all aware of this when we carry a suitcase or shopping with a slightly bent elbow to keep it away from the body. This is performed by static muscle work in the outer range of the flexors of the elbow to hold up the weight and the abductors of the shoulder to hold the arm away from the side, with a long weight lever and gravity pulling the weight of the arm plus the weight in the hand. The working muscles are in every way disadvantaged; they will soon tire and strain may result. Hence the advantage of shopping and luggage trolleys.

When planning any form of muscle work, the type of muscle work and the range in which it will be performed should always be considered, and care taken to vary it at every session. In retraining weak muscles, gentle inner range work, progressing to full range as far as is possible, should be encouraged. Muscles are found in the body in groups. In all types of muscle work, in any range, the opposite group of muscles to that working is always relaxed by the central nervous system.[26]

NERVOUS CONTROL OF MUSCULAR ACTIVITY

Voluntary muscular activity – under the control of the will – is set off from the motor area of the conscious brain.[27] The results of this activity, as registered in skin and fine joint sensation, are sent back to the sensory area of consciousness where they can be appreciated, and are consciously registered. Other joint sensations, tendon feeling and muscular stretch during the activity do *not* reach the consciousness, but go to the spinal cord and centres in the lower, mid and hind brain (cerebellum). From there appropriate orders to help the activity are sent to muscles – either to relax or to contract. These are called 'reflex actions' although they take place in voluntary muscle and are part of the movement pattern. These are not under the control of the will. The cerebellum has overall control of the co-ordination of muscular activity.

It has been known since the middle of the last century that the cortex of the brain controls activity, *not* detailed muscle work. Kinesiologists,[28] anatomists,[29] and physiologists[30] agree on this point. Yet one still sees teachers trying to teach students to perform exact muscle control. Jackson said in 1903 'nervous centres know nothing of muscle; they only know of movement'.[31] Dancers know this instinctively. I want to stress this as I have found it so helpful in trying to teach exercises to different kinds of people. The teacher may think of the muscles requiring training, but must transform the thoughts into directions for movement of the whole body, or the part involved. That movement will have, as its result, the required effect on the muscles in question.

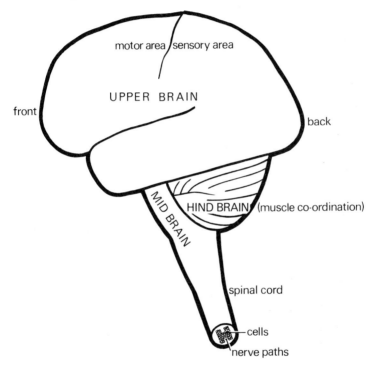

The areas of the brain

Let us take a very simple example. When trying to strengthen the buttock muscles, the old-fashioned way was to say 'pull your bottom tight, try to imagine you are holding a coin between your buttocks'. As there is so much loose fat there, the person can certainly pull this slightly tighter, and if you put your hand under his buttocks as he is sitting you, too, will feel the muscle tighten slightly.

Now what the buttock muscles (gluteus maximus) are really there for, is to pull the thighs backwards at the hip joints and turn them outwards, not lift coins up. Put your hand again under the person's buttocks and tell him to press his thighs onto the seat of the chair, and roll them outwards. You will immediately feel a very strong hard contraction of both his buttock muscles (see p. 131). The person performing the movement will also be easily able to feel the pressure of the skin of his thighs on the chair, and the movements in his hip joints, and so can effectively repeat the performance (skin and joint sensations go directly to the cortex). Or he can perform heel raising, knee bending, with the knees turned outward. Even if he only lowers and raises himself a little way he can feel his joints moving, and if you put your hands on his buttocks, and the front of his thighs, you can feel very strong contractions in both sets of muscles.

Most activities of course have much more complicated muscle work of various kinds, including relaxation of other groups. These can only be taught as a performance, the central nervous system programming the muscle work desired.

Patterns of movement

Patterns of movement is the term given to any activity, whether an apparently simple one like a child sucking his thumb or the amazingly complex one of playing any ball game, where every part of the body is involved. We learn patterns of movement by doing and so we gradually build up a large repertoire of performances. The first activity after birth is based on a reflex that takes the hand to the mouth and upon this the child gradually builds up his knowledge of shape, size, roughness, smoothness, texture, etc. by mouthing and savouring everything within reach. Voluntary movements begin to take shape as his desires increase – 'I want to shake the rattle' – and so for the rest of life, all activities will be a mixture of these two, reflex and voluntary.

The result of voluntary movement – a pattern – is stored in the sensory area of the brain. This final result is called an Engram. Muscular patterns of great complexity and rapidity such as sports, typing, or dancing, can be registered in the sensory area and finally stored in the motor area.[32] Nowadays the sensory and motor areas are believed to be so closely linked that they are sometimes called the senso-motor area.

It is not any old practice that makes perfect, but perfect practice that makes perfect. When we are teaching movement we must remember that the blueprint of it is being laid down in the brain. Mistakes should be eradicated as soon as possible, otherwise they may become permanent. Always remember it is feeling in joints and skin only which informs our consciousness (cortex), while other parts of the pattern go on as reflex activity.

> A centipede was happy quite
> Until a toad in fun,
> Said, 'Pray which leg goes after which?'
> Which worked its mind to such a pitch
> It lay demented in the ditch
> Considering how to run.

This old tongue-twister is very sound modern applied physiology of pattern of movement.[33] Athletes who visualize the performance but not how to do it are the more efficient.[34] Likewise, mirrors in a dance studio are important in helping the dancers to transfer the visual 'shapes' of their performance to the movement memory in the brain. I once heard a harmonica player say, 'When I have a very fast complicated passage to play, as well as breathing in and out by my mouth, I expel the surplus air through my nose. Don't ask me how I do it. I don't know. It just happens.' A dancer said, 'I don't know the steps of the dance, but my feet do.'

Of course both voluntary and reflex actions are taking place alongside each other in complicated muscular patterns. It is the voluntary movements of the pattern, however, that our cortex, in other words our will, can control, and therefore if we pick these out and practise them, our skill will improve with repetition. The reflex movements accompanying the voluntary ones will look after themselves. Repetition is the great secret for success, to allow the whole co-ordinated performance to become smooth and satisfactory. Sir Charles Sherrington, one of the first modern physiologists, said, 'Habit arises always in conscious action; reflex behaviour never arises in conscious action. Habit is always acquired behaviour, reflex behaviour is always inherent and innately given. Habit is not to be confounded with reflex action.'[35]

ASSOCIATED MOVEMENTS

There are many movements that associate in different joints to achieve a chosen result: flexion of the elbow goes with extension of the shoulder, and flexion of the shoulder goes with extension of the elbow. This is often known as the 'sawing reflex'. If you now pretend you are sawing wood, you will find yourself performing it. You will probably be able to find numerous examples of these yourself. They happen because the cortex has given an order for a performance and the muscle association is worked out to get the desired result.

Chemical changes as muscles work

As well as physical changes when muscles work, there are chemical changes within the muscles and in the blood supplying them and leaving them.[36] In every type of muscle work muscles use up the glycogen (sugar) which is stored within the muscle tissue. They also use oxygen from the blood, give off carbon dioxide and lactic acid as waste products, and create heat. If the blood supply through the muscle is flowing well, it brings fresh supplies of glucose (sugar) and oxygen continuously and the waste products are easily carried away in the fluid (tissue fluid) in which all the cells of the body are bathed. This explains why sugar is used up during exercise and why exercise is slimming. The blood brings fresh supplies of energy out of other stores of the body, including fat deposits.

The using up of the oxygen by the muscles and its replenishment from the increased breathing is the 'aerobic process' which is such a feature of well-planned exercise, recommended by physiologists, and experienced exercise teachers. Now when muscles change their length while working, they produce a good pumping action, as do the moving joints, on the small blood vessels (capillaries) and veins. This is especially true of full range movements. Work without movement (isometric, i.e. static) does not have this benign pumping action on the blood and tissue fluid, because the increased muscle bulk bunches up, presses on the smaller blood vessels and impedes the flow of these fluids. It is for this reason that 'isometrics' – the system of working muscles against immovable objects: a desk for the hands, the floor for the leg work, etc. – should be used with caution and intermingled with other freely moving exercises (concentric and eccentric, i.e. isotonic). Isometrics may increase muscle bulk, but if the contraction is sustained for too long at a time the muscles become depleted of oxygen and glycogen and sodden with their own waste products, lactic acid, etc., and will eventually stop working.

As exercise proceeds, blood is hastened back to the heart by the squeezing of the muscles on the capillaries and veins, and by the joints pumping blood onwards. This increased blood flow into the heart causes it to beat more strongly and more blood is pumped out into the arteries, causing a momentary rise in blood pressure. This maintains the blood supply to the lungs and working muscles. Thus the body systems work together; this reinforces the benefit of aerobic conditioning exercises for the heart, lungs and whole body.[37]

Oxygen and heat

As you exercise increased respiration in the lungs is dealing with the increased need for oxygen and for disposal of carbon dioxide.[38] The respiratory centre looks after these requirements, being kept informed by the cortex and working muscles and also by the rise of carbon dioxide in the blood (see p. 72). During the aerobic or oxygen consuming process, heat is given off, more by isometric (static) work and less by isotonic. The body temperature tends to rise. This, however, is taken care of by the regulating centre in the lower brain and then by the system of profit-and-loss which controls body temperature. We are lucky in that we are not like lizards and other reptiles who have to depend on the sun and outside heating: we make our own by cellular activity of all kinds, and it is carried around the body by our warmed blood. This is the profit side.

The loss side is achieved by everything that leaves our bodies, including the damp, warm air from our lungs. Fluid is always being given off by the skin. If this is not sufficient for body temperature loss, then sweating begins. The evaporation of the sweat by the body heat causes the loss of extra heat and the temperature is kept normal. This is why during exercise one should wear cotton or wool next to the skin as these absorb sweat, rather than man-made fibres which do not. It also explains why exercise is difficult in humid conditions, when the air is already so full of fluid that it cannot absorb the evaporated sweat.

OXYGEN DEBT AND SECOND WIND

During exercise the body is capable of incurring an 'oxygen debt'.[39] This means that exercise may continue although the supply of oxygen is not keeping pace with the amount being used in the muscles, in spite of increased respiration both in depth and rate, in that order. After the exercise is finished the respiration continues at the same increased rate until the oxygen debt has been paid off. We have all experienced this after running for a bus, when we have found ourselves panting although we are safely sitting inside it. We have all seen television pictures of athletes running, and then gasping for breath after finishing the race. The capacity to incur an oxygen debt, and deal with it without general collapse, is part of the make-up of a naturally efficient athlete. And it can be improved by training. It is also one of the assets available to those who look after their general health, and who include some form of exercise as a daily regime. Experts say we should get breathless by exercise, while still being able to talk, once a day.

Second wind is the sensation of renewed capability which often overtakes someone who has been exercising strongly, and who up to that moment has been feeling increasing exhaustion. The physiological explanation is not really clear, but it is generally believed that the exhaustion is caused by a build-up of waste products in the working muscles. Then as the increased breathing and blood supply induced by carrying on the activity deal with these, relief ensues. A stronger heart beat due to the blood pouring rapidly into it from the two great veins (upper and lower vena cava) helps greatly. Probably capacity for carrying oxygen debt is also involved. In other words good training brings good results for the whole body.[40]

NERVE–MUSCLE TIREDNESS

Some people complain of being 'always tired'. It is not necessarily muscular fatigue and can have many causes from specific illness to boredom, or tension.[41] If the doctor has ruled out illness it may indicate a need for a healthy training programme.

It is essential for working muscles to have a free flow of blood through them to bring the vital oxygen and to dispose of muscular waste products. If this flow is lessened for any reason, e.g. inflammation, swelling, varicose veins, any exercise should be suitably curtailed. In the normal person, exercise encourages blood flow and by gradually increasing it, more activity becomes possible without fatigue.

Research has shown that in the combination of nerves and muscle, the muscle fibres and nerve fibre are tireless. The junction of the nerve into the muscle and the nerve cell itself, however, are capable of exhaustion. It therefore appears sensible that the more complicated the neuromuscular skill to be learned, the more frequently should rests be given. Little and often is a very good rule for efficient practice.

SLIMMING AND EXERCISE

Activity, coupled with a suitable diet for the age of the person and amount of work done, gets rid of fat. But one can be deceived by the weight on the dial after sensible dieting and exercise. We may be swapping fat for stronger muscles, and the weight may not get less as we had hoped. But we have certainly gained better health by exchanging fat for more efficient muscle fibres. The reverse is also true. Our weight may remain the same as we lose muscle bulk but gain fat, by exercising less and eating more calories than we are using up. The things that matter are body shape, body feeling and performance.[42] A suitable mixed diet containing protein, fats, carbohydrates, vitamins, minerals and water is essential for any muscular activity. So please don't try to become strong and beautiful with a fad diet and massive exercise, all at the same time. You won't succeed.

Summary

This discussion suggests that in learning any skill involving muscle control, from jogging to dancing, or any sport, you apply this knowledge to your own chosen activity.[43]

a. Choose an activity that really fits in with your way of life, and go on to a variety of others.

b. Review your diet for adequate balanced requirements, weighing yourself and counting calories if necessary.

c. Begin activity gently and build up gradually, monitoring your pulse rate if necessary.

d. Develop a mental picture of what you want to achieve in your chosen activity, wholly and in parts, and practise the activity both wholly and in parts.

e. Do not attempt to register muscle work as you practise. Register joint activity and skin sensitivity, and body shape as you move.

f. Practise frequently, not being put off by lack of achievement. Give nerve controls time to learn the pattern for success.

g. Have short sharp bouts of activity interspersed with adequate periods of rest, and change of occupation.

h. Enjoy what you are doing and stop when you get bored or annoyed, and try again later.

i. Get yourself comfortably breathless by exercise, while still able to talk, once a day. This stimulates breathing capacity.

j. Continually review your picture of what you are trying to achieve by watching top-class performers, by being clearly taught, and by experiencing success.

k. Continue practice with only the final clear picture of the activity in mind, making no attempt to direct each single part of it.

l. Practise relaxation (see p. 167) as well as activity, as this is a rule of the body. Remember, if you live 100 years, your heart will have rested more than 50 years.

m. Discontinue all exercise during any acute infections or when overtired. If you have any doubt about your general fitness for exercise, consult your doctor.

3. Bony boxes, muscular boxes, and how they work

I have tried to show in the previous chapter that the functioning of the body is very much interrelated in all its parts, and indeed, with the world in which it finds itself. Students of any kind of kinesiology, or movement training, whether medical, dancing, exercise, etc., learn the nine systems of the body: bony, muscular, nervous, circulatory, digestive, excretory, respiratory, glandular and reproductive. They are sometimes inclined to leave them in these compartments but the parts of the body do not function in isolation, they perform as an integrated whole. It is important to remember this, or we may sometimes cause more damage to the whole person by exercise, than we do good to the local part. Simply clenching the fists puts blood pressure up; prolonged deep breathing may cause fainting; unsuitable abdominal exercise may cause spinal damage or a hernia. Exercise, circulation of blood, breathing, and effects upon abdominal contents are all closely linked.[1] This is why at this point, I want to go deeper into the area of the trunk, i.e. chest (thorax) and abdomen. Also because the abdominal area is the one that everyone wants to reduce in size. At least that is our experience. If someone asks for help in getting fit, and getting rid of extra fat, they usually pat their tummies and say 'especially here'.

The chest

In the body, the more valuable an organ is, the more safely it is stowed away. The most important organs, the brain and spinal cord, are enclosed in very safe bony boxes, the skull and vertebral spinal column. The organs next in order of importance are the heart, lungs and the great blood vessels. These are enclosed in a box, the chest (thorax), which is partly bone and partly muscle. The bones are the twelve vertebrae (spinal column) at the back, the twelve pairs of ribs attached on either side of the vertebrae at the back, and coming round to form the sides and front, eventually attaching to the breastbone (sternum) centre front, by means of movable cartilage (see picture skeleton). The muscle layers are outside the ribs, between them, and inside them. The precious heart and lungs are protected and helped to function by this arrangement of bones, joints, and muscles.

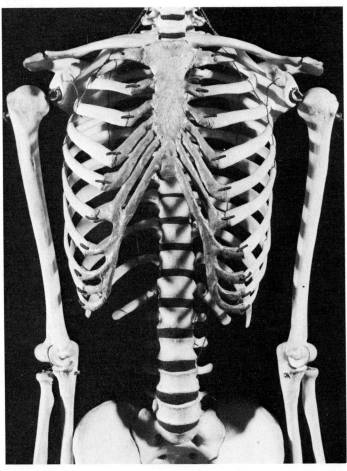

Notice: 1) attachment of collar bones to breast-bone and shoulder blades to collar bones, arms suspended below by loose shoulder joints 2) upper ribs almost horizontal and capable of only slight movement, lower ribs oblique and capable of much fibrous movement 3) each successive rib wider than one above therefore increase of chest width as they are raised when breathing in 4) joint two-thirds of the way up the breast-bone allows much movement during breathing. (Photo: Royal College of Surgeons)

The abdomen

The other bony–muscular box is the abdominal cavity, entirely surrounded by muscle: diaphragm above, pelvic floor below, and abdominal muscles all around. As to bones, there are five vertebrae at the back, and the pelvis below and partly behind.

If you look at the lower part of someone's abdomen from the front, you are not gazing at a bony wall but at a bony rim below, and at a fatty and muscular wall above. Immediately behind are the abdominal and pelvic contents, pressing against the wall. The stomach and intestines have varying amounts of food, fluids, and air inside. Imagine, for example, the quick alteration of bulk inside a beer drinker, who may swallow several pints of beer in a short time, or indeed inside any of us after any large meal. Urine is manufactured continuously by the kidneys as they clean the blood. It immediately flows downwards in two tubes (ureters), one from each kidney, into the bladder, where it collects till it is convenient to discharge it. Then the uterus (womb) may contain nothing and be only about the size of a fist, or it may enlarge to contain a seven- or eight-pound baby, plus a large placenta (one and a half pounds), plus membranes and fluid (about two pounds). It also increases the thickness of its own walls from three ounces to about two pounds during pregnancy.[2] Thus the pressure between the contents and the surrounding abdominal muscles and on the diaphragm above and the pelvic floor below is always varying and sometimes considerable.

The pelvis

What is the pelvis? (see pictures p. 50). It is not really like a 'bony basin' as it is sometimes described 'containing the pelvic organs'. It is more like a knobbly bony saucer, with its flat middle missing, tipped up at the back and down at the front. The lowest vertebral bone (5th lumbar) rests on the centre at the back and the leg bones (right and left femur) are attached at the hip joints at either side. The pelvis is therefore capable of movement at these two hip joints and at the five lumbar joints. It can swivel sideways, or tilt more up in front, or drop further down in front. Indeed it can be moved around in a circle balanced on the legs, as we have seen belly dancers perform.

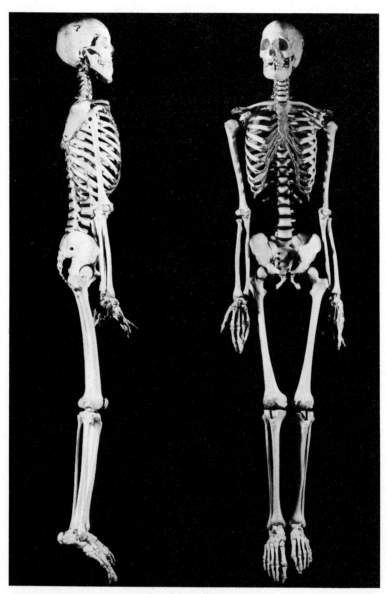

Notice: 1) right shows spinal column straight and left shows curves forwards and backwards 2) delicate neck bones gradually increasing in size downwards 3) slope of ribs downwards and forwards from spinal joints at back to fibrous joints in front 4) right shows saucer-shaped pelvis and left its tilt 5) shoulder girdles perched aslant at top of chest – they carry the arms 6) safe elbow joints but vulnerable knee joints, hence strong thigh muscles 7) feet arched from back to front and side to side. (Photo: Royal College of Surgeons)

The diaphragm

Inside the abdomen the diaphragm is like a circular tent forming a domed ceiling.[3] The top of the tent (central tendon) is not perfectly concave but has a depression in the middle where the heart sits on it, attached by ligaments. This is the 'cardiac depression'. On either side of this depression, bulging upwards, are the right and left domes, at the level of the 8th dorsal vertebra. The diaphragm has two holes in it – one to allow the large vein (inf. vena cava) to convey blood to the heart from the lower half of the body[4] and one to allow the food pipe (oesophagus) to make its way through from above, down to the stomach.[5] The aorta (the largest artery leaving the heart) passes downwards behind the diaphragm in a space just in front of the spinal column, carrying blood to the lower part of the body.

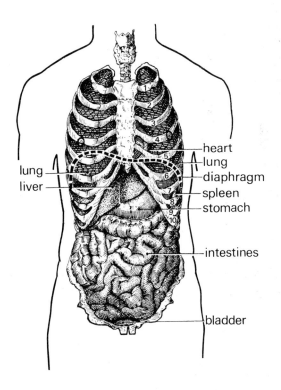

lung
liver

heart
lung
diaphragm
spleen
stomach

intestines

bladder

Abdominal contents

People sometimes speak of the diaphragm as though it were a flat ceiling above the abdomen, about the level of the lower ribs, all the abdominal organs being below, and all the thoracic contents above. The truth is that the biggest abdominal organ, the liver, is entirely enclosed by ribs, presumably for safety, on your right side, and reaches across to the fourth rib interspace on the left, with the arch of the diaphragm resting on the curved upper surface, at the level of the 8th dorsal vertebra (see picture). The stomach in front, the kidneys at the back, and the spleen at the left side, are all enclosed by the lower ribs and lie just under the diaphragm.[6]

Pressure outside and inside

We have already seen how overstuffed the abdomen can be (p. 49). By comparison the chest is underfurnished. The pressure of the atmosphere on every object in the world is fourteen pounds per square inch. But due to their structure and contents, the pressure inside the chest is always less than atmospheric pressure, and that inside the abdomen is always more than atmospheric pressure. Thus if you cut open the chest the contents would fall in, i.e. the lung would collapse. If you cut open the abdominal muscle wall, the guts would protrude. It is like an overstuffed suitcase and we all know what happens to that if the lid bursts open. The negative (minus) pressure in the chest and the positive (plus) pressure in the abdomen is important for us on two counts.

Firstly, the difference in pressure between the top and lower halves of your trunk plays a part in your circulatory system. Since fluid will always flow from an area of high pressure to one of lower pressure, it is one of the main reasons for the flow of blood upwards to the heart. This rate of inflow then determines the output of blood from heart to lungs, and from heart into the aorta, which in turn carries the oxygen-laden blood all over the body. Exercise depends for its aerobic value (see p. 79) on the consumption of oxygen in the working muscles and its replenishment from the lungs. When muscles are working, they use up oxygen and give off carbon dioxide. They also mechanically hasten the return of the blood in the veins towards the heart and so to the lungs. It is only when the blood reaches the lungs that the oxygen can be replenished and the carbon dioxide disposed of. The more blood going through the lungs, the more efficient they become.

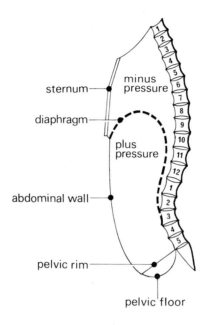

Secondly, the breath should never be held during abdominal exercises as this static contraction of the diaphragm plus the contracting tummy muscles puts up the abdominal pressure very much and may strain the pelvic floor. Any movement of arm or trunk causes a rise in pressure. This pressure can rise four to six times as much and always seeks out the weakest area.[7] In women with a weak pelvic floor, this may cause an embarrassing issue of urine, or even muscular damage. The breath should always be expelled gently during the abdominal contraction, thus lessening the abdominal plus pressure and assisting the shortening of the working muscles.

Pelvic floor muscles and exercises

Due to our upright posture and the forward tilt of our pelvis the pelvic floor is practically parallel with the ground, sweeping upwards somewhat at the back. It is composed of several muscles, variously named (levator ani). [8] There are two identical sets of muscles growing from the inside of either side of the pelvis and the fibrous material (fascia) which covers other muscles. The two sides meet in midline around and in front of the back passage to form a gutter, but in the front around the vagina and urethra there is a narrow gap in the muscles. This gap gets wider when the muscles are weak.

When the pelvic floor muscles contract the edges come together, lift and are flattened. Conversely sudden increases of pressure in the abdomen caused by the diaphragm contracting when sneezing or coughing, causes the pelvic floor to bulge down and become a deeper gutter shape.

The pelvic floor is perforated by the back passage (anus) to allow residue from the bowel to be discharged, and at the front is the urethra for the passage of urine. In women the vagina lies between these two passages.

Every woman should learn how to control her pelvic floor. As it is made of exactly the same kind of muscle as that in the arms and legs and abdominal muscles, it is capable of contracting when told to perform a function. This function is to close the gap in the muscles and raise the pelvic floor. There is a lot of a loose kind of fat around the contents of the pelvic floor, and it is in here and in the skin covering, that nerves provide the sensation of squeezing and lifting.

Strong resilient pelvic floor muscles are necessary to resist the pull of gravity from below and the abdominal organs pressing down from above. They also enhance the pleasure of sexual intercourse for both partners and aid the safe delivery of a baby, as well as helping to restore the uterus and other soft parts to their correct positions after delivery.

To strengthen the pelvic floor muscles at any age there are two exercises to perform.

1. Each time you empty your bladder stop and start the flow of urine two or three times – you will feel the squeeze and lift underneath as you do this.
2. When sitting, standing or lying down practise squeezing the anus closed, then make the squeezing pass forward to the vagina and urethra so that the loose tissue and skin feels drawn upwards into yourself. Count four and let go slowly. Repeat four times. Try to practise this at least once each hour.

Do not pull the buttocks together or squeeze the thighs closed as you may mistake the wrong feeling for the correct one. This used to be taught when false modesty prevented mention of the pelvic floor, which was rather foolish and unhelpful. Instead, concentrate on the exact area you are trying to move. This is possible because of the unique formation and function of the pelvic floor, which has no joint to work upon, but instead tightens around all its canals and their orifices, rather like pursing up the mouth. It also squeezes and lifts its own special loose fascia upwards. The sensitive skin and the movement of the fascia will help you to register the result of your efforts.

If you persevere, practising about five lifting squeezes every half hour or hour, as may be convenient, you will gradually develop a strong pelvic floor and may prevent many gynaecological difficulties in later life. It is a good exercise to do at a bus stop or when washing up or feeding a baby. No-one watching will know what you are doing, but you will benefit considerably. During a coughing fit you should also try to contract the pelvic floor, otherwise the sudden repeated rise in abdominal pressure caused by diaphragmatic activity puts strain on it and may cause leakage of urine. (See remarks on dangers of double leg lifting, p. 61.)

Abdominal muscles and exercises

If you look at your naked body sideways in a long glass you will see that your abdomen bulges forward. This is because everyone has two layers of fat there. The muscle layer is sandwiched between the fatty ones. The first layer of fat is immediately under the skin; just below lies the muscle layer, then another layer of fat and just under that a layer of lining (peritoneum). Under this are the intestines padded by fat.[9] Women have thicker fat deposits in the abdomen than men, as they have all over the body (see p. 20.)

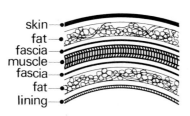

skin
fat
fascia
muscle
fascia
fat
lining

If you want to keep that bulge under control, it helps to realize what is going on in there, and that these abdominal muscles are always weighed down by the two fat deposits, outer and inner, each time they try to work.

The correct name for the abdominal sheet of muscle is the antero-lateral abdominal wall. This is really a very helpful one because it reminds us that it covers the entire front (antero) from ribs to pelvis, and wraps completely around each side (lateral), reaching thick fibrous layers (fascia) at the back where it is attached to the vertebrae of the spinal column. So when we refer to 'the tummy muscles' we do them less than justice – but it is a handy term.

If you imagine a straight line from the tip of the breast-bone down to the top of the pelvic bone below, there would be an identical set of abdominal muscles on either side. This line is called the *linea alba* (white line) and each set of muscles, right and left, attach into it. You may have seen a slightly discoloured brownish stripe vertically down the middle of the abdomen after pregnancy, over the white line, if there has been extra stretching of the abdominal muscles.

In each set of muscles there are three layers (external oblique, internal oblique and transversalis). None of these layers or sheets completely covers the area, but their fibres fan out in varying directions spreading across their side of the abdomen; so that together, when they meet at the midline in front, they practically make a complete cover. They have of course fascial layers between them and fascia into which they attach at the back, in front, above and below. There is an extra muscle reinforcement (rectus abdominus) in front lying on each side of the midline running from the breast-bone and ribs above on either side to the pelvis below. The 'tummy muscles' are in fact a closely knit series of muscle layers whose fibres, plus their attaching fascia, run in all directions covering the whole circumference of the abdominal pelvic cavity.[10] But we have not yet finished surrounding the abdominal cavity with muscle. There is also an abdominal wall of muscle at the back. This posterior group of muscles lies inside the circumference of the abdominal muscles already described. The direction of the group (iliopsoas and quadratus) is vertical and it will therefore work with the straight side fibres of the other abdominal muscles.

The massive sheet of abdominal muscle does not work by individual muscle but by direction of its fibres, irrespective of single muscles. To understand this you may find the following helpful. Imagine you have draped a Union Jack flag right across your tummy, having its middle white line dead centre. Attach it to the ribs above, the pelvis below, and right round each side to the spinal column at the back. If you now think of each colour in the Union Jack shortening in turn you will know the actions of the abdominal muscles.

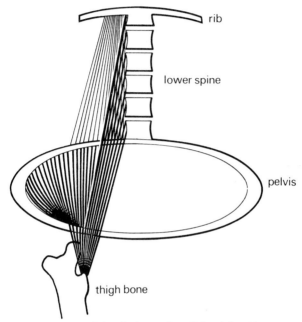

Posterior abdominal muscles of the right side

The straight up-and-down fibres in front on both sides of the white line will either bring the chest towards the pelvis, as in lying, and forward bending, or the pelvis towards the chest as in pelvic tilting (see pp. 127, and 153). The straight fibres at the sides will work with the straight fibres of back muscles and posterior abdominal muscles on the same side to side bend the chest towards the pelvis (side flexion) or pelvis towards the chest (pelvis side lifting). See exercises on pp. 121, 155.

The oblique fibres running diagonally from the right side of chest to the left side of pelvis, right across the white line, will rotate the right side of the chest towards the left side of the pelvis or the left side of pelvis to the right side of chest, and the opposite diagonal fibres will do the same in the opposite directions (trunk rotations, see exercises on pp. 123, 125). All the fibres of the entire muscular sheet will work together to compress, flatten and narrow the whole area in any expulsive effort upwards or downwards (sneezing, coughing, vomiting, passing urine or faeces or delivering a baby). This they do by increasing the plus pressure in the abdominal cavity. It is usually associated with a strong diaphragmatic contraction which assists the expulsion by also increasing the plus pressure from above.

We want to tighten up our 'tummy muscles' and reduce that local burden of two layers of fat; in other words to make our tummies smaller and neater by exercise. To train this sheet of muscle effectively, make it stronger and tighter and get rid of the local fat, we always need four exercises, because of the four main directions of the fibres.

1. Straight up and down in front
2. Straight up and down at each side
3. Oblique in opposite directions in front and around sides
4. Compression, i.e. narrowing in all directions

Only by doing all four movements will we have exercised the abdominal muscles fully, owing to their unique arrangement.

In conclusion, what everyone wants are shorter, stronger, less fatty abdominal muscles, not bulkier ones strong as iron bars, unless we are professional weight-lifters. A neater, smaller outline is what most people crave, so all exercise of the abdominal muscles should finally aim at inner range, concentric (p. 34), shortening movements, associated with an easy outward breath, to keep down the abdominal pressure.

The back and exercises

BACK JOINTS AND HIP JOINTS

The joints at which the movements take place are the spinal joints between each vertebra and sometimes also the hip joints. The shape of the joints will determine where the action actually takes place. Forward bending takes place in all joints, although very little in the upper back. There is practically no side bending in the upper back but a great deal in the lower back and in the neck. There is no rotation in the lower back but plenty in the neck, upper back and hips.[11] Let us therefore consider briefly the structure of the back muscles.

BACK MUSCLES

Again we find the muscles are arranged in layers, none of which completely covers the back.[12] The topmost layers are the widest; they then become smaller the deeper they lie. The muscles under the skin and outer layer of fat are the largest; just two cover the whole back. The upper one (trapezius), moves the head, the neck, the shoulder girdles, and the spine – once again we see the wonderful versatility of muscles (see exercises on pp. 99, 101). The other large muscle (latissimus dorsi) lower down the back will extend the spine backwards and also take the arm back (see exercise on p. 103). It will help in side bending and as some of its fibres lie in an oblique direction, it can help in rotation of the trunk.

Under these two muscles are layers of smaller muscles all running in varying directions, of different shapes and sizes and in turn moving the shoulder blades, both outwards and inwards (serratus anterior, rhomboids) and also upwards (levator anguli scapulae); enlarging the chest by pulling on the ribs (serratus posterior superior and inferior); and extending the whole of the spinal column and head (erector spinae). This last long strong muscle of many segments is also a strong side flexor. Then deep under all this are tiny muscles crossing between adjacent or near vertebrae and in turn running in different directions (rotatores, etc.). They assist the larger stronger muscles in appropriate movements, depending on the direction of their fibres and angle of pull.

Here we are again with different muscles all ready to shorten in many directions, in fact in all directions except when we bend quickly forward. They will work with the abdominal muscles in any way they can to perform the movements demanded; if they are not assisting they will be relaxed. So let us remember once again that the body works in unison for function, that is for action, the muscle groups involved in various ways being selected and controlled by the central nervous system, not the conscious brain.

Since the orders we give to our bodies from our conscious brain are for actions, not exact muscular work (see p. 38), all muscles that can assist in the project will do so. If we say 'bend to the side' the straight side fibres of the front abdominal muscles, and the post abdominal muscles, as we have seen, as well as the back muscles on that side, will join in if their fibres run in a suitable direction. The same is true of rotation. If we say 'twist to the right or left', all the oblique fibres that can be of assistance will be working, whether of the abdominal muscles or the ones on the back. Your teacher, when giving exercises to a class, should be aware of this. He or she must know how to get the class to use the muscles previously selected for strengthening or relaxation, not by trying to direct those specific muscles, but by giving exact orders for a movement which they know will cause the result they want. The same applies to the person exercising alone. Let us take an example. If the teacher has asked for side bending of the trunk in which the class is expected to use the side flexors, i.e. straight fibres of the trunk (abdominal and back muscles), a very wary eye must be kept on the class to see that they really do bend sideways and not arch back as they do so. If they do arch back, they are using mostly back muscles. Equally they must not bend forwards or they will be using mostly abdominal muscles. Some people may twist instead of bending sideways, thus using more oblique fibres than the selected straight side ones, and as we have seen, getting movement in a different area of the spine.

Again, if the teacher wants to concentrate on the oblique fibres, the class should perform a true rotation, keeping either the pelvis fixed or the chest fixed as they do so. As the oblique fibres form the strongest part of the abdominal muscular corset, they should be particularly well exercised.

Precautions and dangers

All teachers of exercise should be aware of the weak points in the abdomen and back and of all the dangers of increasing abdominal pressure.[13]

HERNIA

There is always a danger of rupture (hernia) if strong abdominal contractions are encouraged without due care in training. The old and the weak are especially vulnerable if the abdominal muscles have been allowed to become very slack (see p. 13). Equally, holding your breath when bending forwards to lift objects is an easy way to a rupture. Breathe out and bend your hips and knees as you lift that box. Keep your back straight.

This can be caused by a sudden forward bending of the trunk, especially if the breath is held. What happens is that the abdominal pressure is suddenly increased and if all the trunk muscles, back and front, are not in good condition, something gives way. You may damage a ligament, a disc, a bone, or tear a muscle (see p. 30). Prevent it by gradual training of all the trunk muscles, and mobilization of all the vertebral joints, before any strong forward bending is attempted. No-one should ever bend forward to pick up a heavy object. Instead the back should be kept straight, the breath should not be held, and the object reached by bending the hips and knees. Then keep the object close to the body when rising up. This technique is now becoming fairly well known. But people forget.

Pushing a broken-down car is a popular sport in winter. It is dangerous if performed facing the car with two extended arms touching it, the head and back rounded forward, and the breath held; especially so if the feet are slipping on icy ground. One should put one's back towards the car with the hands low down, pressing palms against it and getting the feet as near to the car as possible. Then heave backwards, taking the weight from the hips, with a straight back so that the large back and buttock muscles are taking the strain, doing the work, and also protecting the smaller deeper muscles and bones.

DOUBLE LEG RAISING

I have seen so many women, young and old, who have been damaged by attempting to perform this exercise. There is an idea abroad that if any exercise be difficult or even painful, it must therefore be doing you good. This is not true. A well-chosen and well-performed exercise will always be accompanied by a sense of satisfaction and pleasure, and although it may be hard work there will never be any sense of strain. As this exercise is so often advocated for strengthening the tummy muscles, let us go through it in detail, to see why it is not a good idea to perform it, especially for women.

The person lies on the ground and is told to lift both legs, keeping the knees straight and moving from the hips. The working muscles are the flexors of the hips. These muscles are always fairly strong already, as they are used in every step one takes. In any case all flexors in the body, that is to say those that bend up the body towards its centre, tend to be stronger than their opposite groups, the extensors. Therefore there is no need to strengthen this particular group of flexors.

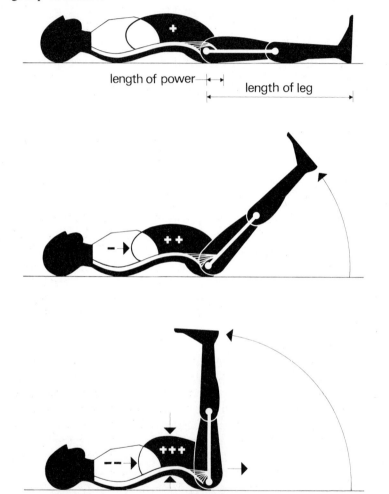

The dangers of double leg raising

The work each group is doing, is equal to the length of each leg multiplied by the weight of each leg (see p. 24). People are apt to think they are simply lifting the weight of their legs, but do remember that every action is governed by the laws of gravity and leverage, in this case third-class leverage. Therefore the flexor muscles are not simply working against the weight of the leg but the weight of the leg *multiplied* by the *length* of the leg. This is about 80 to 85 cms. The length of the lever by which the flexors' power is multiplied is only the distance from the hip joint to the upper part of the femur on the inside (smaller trochanter) to which they attach. This is about 3 to 5 cms. They are therefore working at a great leverage disadvantage (see the picture of hip flexors on p. 57).

What is called reciprocal relaxation (see pp. 40, 167) always takes place in any muscular performance, therefore the extensors of the hips are relaxed by the central nervous system, while the flexors are working. The extensors of the hips are the buttock muscles which are heavily endowed with fat. No woman wants to make these muscles more relaxed, instead she wants to tighten them up and get rid of the surrounding fat.

So now we have this colossal amount of work given to the flexors to do and to the same extent we have weakened the extensors. Remember the plus pressure always present within the abdominal pelvic cavity. The flexors of the hips are attached above to the vertebrae of the low back as well as inside the pelvis (see p. 57) and below near the top end of the thigh bone. As these muscles are having so much difficulty raising the long and heavy legs, the upper end pulls the vertebrae forwards and rolls the pelvis downwards and forwards. This stretches the lower attachments of the abdominal muscles. You may have noticed if you have attempted to do this exercise that your lower back comes off the floor; that is you hollow your back. Even though your teacher tells you not to do so, you cannot avoid it. This is because the spinal joints are being pulled forward as described above. Because the pressure inside the abdomen is always a plus pressure the abdominal wall therefore is distended forwards.

To try to stabilize the moving spinal joints, the abdominal muscles try to work. They have now been pushed into their stretched, outer range position and are trying to work statically. These two conditions are the most difficult for any muscle (see p. 38), and in any re-education programme are only used when the muscle has been given considerable strengthening training.

The abdominal muscles now find themselves very strained and possibly quiver. It is for this reason that people who don't know the anatomy involved, imagine this exercise is 'good for' the abdominal muscles. They mistake strain for healthy activity.

But there is more strain still to come. Because the abdominal muscles are attached to the ribcage above as well as the pelvis below, they tend to pull at the ribcage. To prevent this movement and to stabilize the working abdominal wall the performer automatically holds the breath so that by fixing the diaphragm the ribs may be held firm from inside where the diaphragm attaches.

Often people are told to hold the legs fixed in the air for some time, then to lower them slowly, then to hold them again and to repeat this till they reach the ground. This gives static muscle work to the flexors of the hips followed by eccentric work alternately, into the outer range. This compounds the already overwhelming difficulties.

So here is the situation at the moment. The flexors of the hip are being strengthened; the extensors of the hip are being weakened and the vulnerable area of the low back is being strained. The abdominal muscles are being stretched, and are attempting to work under very difficult conditions. The breath is being held, which is putting up the abdominal pressure from + + to + + +. The whole force is therefore going on to the pelvic floor. The pelvic floor tends to be weak in women through lack of use and is always weaker than in men, thanks to the presence of the vagina and the urethra, the tube leading from the bladder to the outside. This pressure can be very dangerous, especially after the stretching imposed on the pelvic floor during child-birth.

When doing this exercise it is common for women to experience a slight gush of urine due to the sphincter (circular) part of the pelvic floor muscles around the urethra being unable to withstand the increased abdominal pressure. This demonstrates the force thrust downwards on the pelvic floor. Usually the woman is too self-conscious to mention the unpleasant flow to her teacher. This same leaking of urine is found by women in the late ante-natal stage or early post-natal stage, when they cough, as this involves a strong contraction of the diaphragm. The increased abdominal pressure is transferred as force onto the weakened pelvic floor muscles.

The result of this dreadful exercise if persisted in by women, apart from tiring them very much, is to strengthen the flexors of the hips, which is unnecessary, weaken the buttock muscles, stretch and strain their abdominal and pelvic floor muscles, and put great strain on the low back. These joints are already loosened by hormone influence during pregnancy. Grave physical damage may result. This is the reason why I have given so much space to explaining this exercise. Physiotherapists from the obstetric and gynaecological Association of the Chartered Society have been warning against it for years. Clem Thompson in his book *Structural Kinesiology* says 'Leg raising is primarily hip flexion and not abdominal action. Backs may be injured by strenuous and prolonged leg-raising exercises.'[14]

SIT-UPS WITH A STRAIGHT BACK

The exercise of lying flat, possibly with the feet held firmly down, and raising the trunk upwards is really the same exercise as double leg raising. The only difference is that the hip flexors are working in reverse in a way for which they were not designed. The trunk of course is even heavier than the legs to lift and so the strain is greater. This exercise is therefore also unsuitable for women and doubtful for men unless perhaps for the already very fit.

This exercise should not be confused with 'curl-ups', in which the head is curled forward, kept low towards the abdomen and slight bending of the whole spine takes place. The main working muscles are the straight middle fibres of the abdominal muscles plus support from the whole sheet of muscle. If carefully performed this may be a useful exercise as training progresses.

Let us therefore respect this complicated arrangement of bones, muscles, and contents of the whole trunk, so that we may upgrade the muscle control and lubricate the joints safely, without causing harm to them or anything else.

4. Posture and balance, breathing and circulation

'Unto the upright there ariseth light in the darkness'
Psalm 112 v. 4

Posture and balance

The upright posture is called a 'dynamic' one which means that it is a slightly moving, alive, vibrant, changing one, responding all the time, although usually we are totally unaware of it, to all kinds of pressures. The slightest shift of our body weight produces re-actions all over the body to adjust the line and centre of gravity (see p. 21) and keep us upright. We may use body, head, arm, or even leg movements either separately or working together for this purpose like a tight-rope walker. This goes on all the time and of course the more our body keeps aware of pressures and position of joints, and is capable of responding to all kinds of stimuli, the healthier, happier, and safer we are.

Many falls are caused because people no longer have dynamic posture. They have become non-reactive lumps of flesh; one small displacement of their centre of gravity and over they go. If you stay a few weeks in bed and don't do movements to retain your muscular control and skin and joint feelings, when you get up you may well have to cling to furniture as you attempt to walk. I have seen people travel round the room like chimpanzees, using two arms and two legs, instead of human beings, able to stand freely on one leg as we do with every normal step we take.

A young farmer aged twenty-four had the fearful misfortune to have both his arms amputated after they had been caught in some farm machinery.[1] When he was recovering he had to learn to control his balance when standing, all over again; without any arms his centre of gravity was completely altered. Cherish your balance, exercise it daily and always try to improve it: it may save you from a broken leg or a fractured skull one day. Instead of falling when your balance is somewhat disturbed and your line of gravity is going out-side your base, you easily stay upright. Your wonderful body has the mechanism but it is your job to keep it in good order by frequent use. 'Poor posture puts more work on muscle, more strain on ligaments, abnormal strains on bones and may eventually produce deformities. It interferes with respiration, heart action, digestion, and detracts from feelings of self-confidence.'[2]

When a baby is born the spine is curved backwards from head to pelvis. At about six months he or she has developed the forward curve in the neck by moving the head. From about four to nine months the baby can probably sit unsupported and is beginning to develop the lumbar curve forwards; at about ten months to a year and a half he or she walks with a very exaggerated lumbar curve, and the tummy protrudes in consequence.[3]

All this time, by trial and error, the balance mechanism is being developed. Just as control of the mechanism has to be learned, so it can be lost by faulty use, or by lack of use. Muscular weakness, habit, fashion, wrong shoes, pregnancy and a multitude of other reasons, emotional and physical – all can affect balance adversely. Adults may have sway back, forward-thrust pelvis, round shoulders, poking head, and all the other variations of the child's growing programme. They may also develop spinal deformity by habitual wearing of high-heeled shoes, carrying a shoulder bag, or a heavy briefcase. They are not to be blamed, and usually although they may suffer aches and pains they are not really ill, although they may become so if neglected. They have lost the capacity to feel their body shape and often do not know what is the normal standing adult posture. But it can easily be learned. Here is a diagram of the mechanism by which the upright posture of man is maintained whether he is standing, dancing, running, or playing some game requiring control of balance.

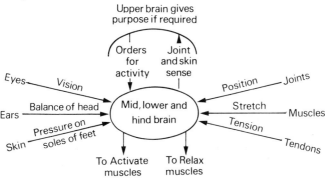

Eyes (sight), ears because of the fluid in the semicircular canals which indicate the position of the head, muscle stretch, joint and tendon sensation, pressure on the soles of feet, all send messages to the spinal cord, middle, low, and hind brain. The incoming messages are co-ordinated and then suitable messages are sent out to the exact muscle pattern that will retain the upright posture or any required balance. The incoming messages do not reach the conscious brain, they are much too quick for that. So they require practice. Only repetition keeps the mechanism performing smoothly. It is quite easy to keep it going, so do try.

Watch a child training his balance when he is learning to walk. No matter how often he falls over, up he gets again till he can control changing his weight from one leg to the other. Then he practises turning, and later he will practise climbing, walking along narrow or high walls. If he has a wise mother she will allow him freedom to do all this natural training, except perhaps for really dangerous balancing, over basement steps, for instance. In fact, if she joins in balancing games, her own muscles all over her body will respond to the stimulation of skin, joints, tendons, muscles, eyes, and ears registering her changes of weight as she sways. This is excellent natural training of body control in response to body sensation. From middle age onwards it is vital to maintain your 'sense of balance' in good trim. Fractures from falls are common in old age and may be prevented by maintaining postural control.

The correct upright posture, first described in 1889, had the line of gravity through the ankle, knee, hip, and shoulder joints to a point just behind the ear.[4] This alignment is still taught by some people but modern ideas are not so rigid. The line is now considered usually to pass in front of the ankles, through the knees and behind the shoulders, up to just behind the ear.[5] See the picture of the skeleton in profile on p. 50. The accepted idea is that good upright posture is one which allows every part of the body to function well. Good health and good posture are reciprocally related – that is each depends upon the other. So what must we do to preserve good posture? Here is a very easy way to register your own posture and therefore to be able to adjust it at will.

Stand with your feet just slightly apart and you will find they naturally turn out very slightly. Now sway gently forwards and you will feel the pressure of your weight on your toes – this is too far forward. Now gently sway backwards and you will feel the pressure going through your heels – which is too far back. Now adjust your weight so that it falls through to your feet just in front of your ankles. This is easy to do and is the position in which your feet are made to receive it. The result is that your weight now goes from the point just in front of your ankles, through your feet, partly downwards at the heel, and partly spread across the middle of your feet onto the toes. This is why the foot is arranged in arches from back to front, and from side to side, so that our weight may spring forward as we walk. It is designed for movement, not like an arch in a building, which is merely for static support.[6] When standing you sway slightly forwards and backwards continuously although you are unaware of it. The sway gives alternate muscle work to the muscles in the front and back of the lower leg, and thus allows them rest periods as well as work periods.[7]

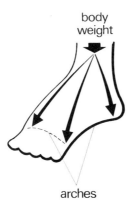

body
weight

arches

Now, keeping your weight in front of your ankles, just gently wiggle your knee-caps up and down; you should find this quite easy. This demonstrates that the knees are not being held in a rigid straight line by the quadriceps muscles in front, which we used to think was the case. They are in fact kept, along with the hips, in an easy position by action of the hamstrings at the back of the thigh which control both joints, knee, and hip.[8]

Now we have reached your pelvis and many people wonder what position it is meant to be in. So try out the four possibilities. Place your hands on the protruding knobs of bone on either side of your tummy, thrust your pelvis forwards, and you will immediately feel that it is out of body alignment. Then thrust it far back, and you will also feel it to be uncomfortable. Now tilt it downwards in front and you will feel your bottom is protruding at the back – obviously wrong. Try reversing the tilt – up in front and so down at the back. This may feel better but still odd and out of balance, so release it and feel the pelvis in balance in mid position so that your weight line (line of gravity) is passing through your knees, and just in front of your ankles.[9]

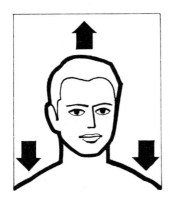

The three-point pull

You are learning to feel your weight and to control its passage through your body. Now from this stable foundation, stretch your spine so that your breast-bone tilts up slightly, carrying your whole chest to a slightly uplifted position. Keep breathing gently, feeling your lower ribs lift up sideways and then drop. Continue this stretch through your neck to your head, keeping your eyes facing forwards and your chin at a right angle to your neck. Your ears should be just above your shoulders. As you stretch the top of your head up, pull your shoulders straight down towards the floor. I call this the three-point pull. Your arms fall easily at your sides. Retain this position without any effort, just conscious of your erect head, your easy breathing, and the slight sway at the ankles. This stretching reduces somewhat the three curves of the spine (see p. 50) which is a very helpful movement to make several times a day for a moment or two, whether you are standing or sitting. When weight is being carried through any curve the brunt of it goes onto the concavity. So by stretching the curve this burden is eased temporarily. This may save ligamentous or bony damage from accumulating. No-one wants osteo-arthritis.

You are now in a corrected balanced standing position with the minimum of muscles working, no undue strain on ligaments or bones, and a helpful position of the chest for easy breathing; the abdominal organs are not cramped while they continue to digest your last meal, and your huge liver gets on with its essential multiple jobs. You will probably feel more alert and happy. Now that you have felt these easy adjustments, try facing a long mirror and repeat them, then stand sideways to the mirror and repeat them. It is quite surprising to watch your shape altering for the better with each small joint control, but do keep on feeling what you are doing. Remember also that you must never hold yourself rigidly. You will become adept at making such small adjustments that no-one else will know that you are doing so. No spectacular heaving up of the chest is necessary, or over-exaggeration of any kind. You simply adjust the way in which your weight passes through your joints. This is easy to do with a little practice. Do keep breathing easily as you make the joint changes, and do not try to retain the corrected position for very long. Learn to take it and leave it, remembering that the natural body sway forwards and backwards, or from side to side, although imperceptible, makes your muscles have bursts of activity automatically.[10] When you feel part of your body sagging, or being distorted, it is good that you should know how to adjust it readily and comfortably.[11] See Corrected Standing p. 165.

There are really no such things as arm exercises, leg exercises, etc., although we use the term, as it is useful to indicate whereabouts the emphasis in each exercise will fall. But the body is not like a jointed doll, made up of separate sections, that you can move quite independently of the rest. Just by raising your arms above your head, your centre of gravity moves upwards and so changes the muscular patterns needed to control your balance. The body is an integrated whole and must be respected as such.

When you are training your posture and balance you may find some part that is difficult to control, e.g. your pelvic balance. Turn to Chapters 6 and 7 and you will find exercises you may care to do which will loosen any joints involved, strengthen weak muscles or stretch shortened ones, and help you get control of the exact area.

Breathing and blood circulation

We are composed of a mass of cells of various types busily working, breaking down and building themselves up. This process is called our metabolism. All cells in the body need oxygen to function and give off carbon dioxide as a waste product. An adult at rest uses about 250 mls of oxygen and produces about 200 mls of carbon dioxide per minute.[12] The blood brings to all body cells the oxygen which it has obtained from the air in the lungs and carries away the carbon dioxide to be disposed of in turn by the lungs. The number of small blood vessels (capillaries) open in the working muscles and the lungs is greatly increased by regular exercise, during which the interchange may be twenty times greater than when the body is at rest.[13]

The amount of carbon dioxide in the blood is the most important among a number of factors that control one's breathing. The other factors can be shown in diagrammatic form:

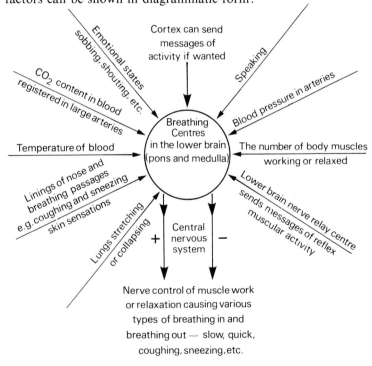

The Many Influences controlling Respiration[14]

The finely tuned nature of respiration control is a fundamental fact that should be appreciated by everyone who attempts to control their own, or anyone else's breathing. The delicate control can be so easily upset by well-meant but clumsy attempts 'to increase the supply of oxygen'. As is plain from the diagram above, there are a great number of 'inputs' to the series of pairs of breathing centres on either side in the low brain which control the type of breathing required.

BREATHING IN

The action of the diaphragm and the muscles between the ribs (external intercostals) increases the size of the chest in three dimensions:

1 vertical
2 from side to side
3 from back to front

Diaphragm. We know the diaphragm has two domes in its upper curve. These descend about 2 or 3 cms and, with the whole central tendon, are then resting on the liver. In this way, the vertical measurement of the chest is increased. The diaphragm then pulls on the lower ribs via their attachments to it on the inside. The ribs, due to their bent and curved shape, and to the angle of their joints, perform a curved movement outwards and upwards. This is aptly described as a 'bucket-handle movement' and increases the sideways size of the chest, because each rib is wider than the one immediately above, which it replaces as they rise.

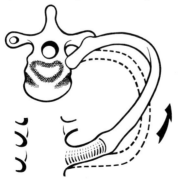

The 'bucket-handle' movement of the ribs

External intercostal muscles help the diaphragm to haul out the lower ribs. They are attached between the ribs, running diagonally downwards towards the midline, and thus can pull them both upwards and outwards. The true bucket handle movement gradually increases in the six lower pairs of ribs. This causes a much enlarged lower chest, the sideways measurement increasing the lower we look.[15]

As the ribs are lifted upwards they prod finally on the breast-bone (sternum) in front, forcing the lower two-thirds of it gently forwards. The upper part is held by the first rib on either side. We have now a bigger measurement in the chest from front to back.

Lining the ribs there is a double layer of fine fibrous tissue (pleurae) with a small amount of fluid between the layers so that they glide easily on each other. The outer layer is attached to the ribs and the inner layer to the lungs, so when the chest expands it pulls the lungs out with it.

We know that the pressure inside the chest is always less than the atmosphere, i.e. it is negative (p. 52). This increase in size means that it is now *more* negative. Since nature abhors a vacuum and since the atmospheric pressure outside is now much greater than within the chest, air from outside pours down the breathing passages into the expanding lungs and will fill them where they are most distended. As we have seen, this is in the lower areas and it is here therefore that most ventilation takes place.[16] If you put your hand on the thorax of any resting cat or dog which is fully grown, you will feel this gentle continuous rib movement. You can even see it when they lie asleep. Don't, however, watch or feel a young child for information about the adult chest. At birth the ribs are in a horizontal position and breathing is by a piston action of the diaphragm and said to be abdominal in type. It is not until the seventh year that respiration is shared by the ribs.[17]

BREATHING OUT

Breathing out (expiration) is entirely passive. Information reaches the breathing centres in the low brain that carbon dioxide content in the blood is decreasing, and that the elastic lung walls are being stretched somewhat. The breathing centres then tell the inspiratory muscles via their central nervous system nerves to relax. The diaphragm relaxes and so the domes rise up, and the plus pressure in the abdomen, aided by the tautness of the abdominal wall, causes the abdominal contents to be pressed up against the underside of the diaphragm. This pressure on the bases of the lungs helps to press air out. Also when the intercostal muscles between the ribs, and the diaphragm both relax, the ribs fall downwards and inwards, the breast-bone falls backwards, and all this pressure around the lungs helps to squeeze out more air. The lungs themselves also have 'elastic recoil' after being distended by the air. If the lungs (alveoli) were opened up and spread out they would cover a tennis court, i.e. about seventy square metres or some forty times the surface area of the skin of the entire body.[18] So you have plenty of capacity, if you use it properly.

We never of course completely empty our lungs of air until we exhale our last breath on earth, so it is unnecessary to encourage people to 'empty that stale air at the base of the lungs by breathing out fully' as we often hear people being exhorted to do. The base of the lungs is where most ventilation takes place. The chest isn't like a pot of coffee with the grounds falling to the bottom. In fact the blood passes through the whole lung system in half a second and therefore different blood is continuously available for the interchange of oxygen and carbon dioxide.[19] The blood of course is sent to the lungs for this refreshment by the contractions of the heart. We must remember the heart beats, i.e. contracts, about seventy-two times per minute in the average adult.

The amount of work the heart does is in direct relation to the amount of blood entering from the veins. It forces out exactly the same quantity into the lungs (by the right ventricle) and into the aorta (by the left ventricle) as it has received from the veins. Hence the importance of regular exercise and increased breathing to maintain a resilient, strongly beating heart. It is contraction of muscle, movements of joints, and the difference between the plus pressure in the abdomen and minus pressure in the chest that pushes the blood onwards in the veins, on its return journey to the heart. As training continues, the heart thickens and so strengthens to do the increased work and its rate slows as its efficiency improves.[20]

FORCED BREATHING

The cortex of the brain has overall control of movements of the body, and so it is possible to increase the amount of air breathed in or breathed out by orders from the cortex for increased activity.[21]

Forced inspiration. A normal inward breath is performed by the diaphragm and the muscles between the ribs (external intercostals), but a forced inspiration can be carried out by all muscles which have any attachment to the ribs, whether in the neck, arms, back, or chest. It depends on how much the inspiration is forced as to how many muscles are used. Sometimes, as in asthma, the person clasps his or her hands together or holds onto any furniture handy, such as a table, to fix the arms and shoulder girdles and so give the muscles attached there more power to pull out the chest wall. In forced inspiration about 2,500 to 3,000 mls more air can enter the lungs (inspiratory reserve air).

Forced expiration. The main muscles working to force air out of the lungs are the abdominal muscles which, by shortening inwards, increase the abdominal plus pressure and thus insist on the domes of the diaphragm rising as high as possible (8th dorsal vertebra). Because the abdominal muscles are attached to the ribs, they also pull them downwards and inwards when they contract. All muscles that can diminish the chest size in its three dimensions will work, and so the air is pushed out into the atmosphere. The amount of air capable of being expelled by forced expiration is about 1,000 to 1,500 mls (expiratory reserve air). There is always a reserve of air in the lungs throughout life of about 1,500 mls (residual air). This is being mixed and refreshed with every breath in and out.[22]

INTERFERING WITH THE BREATHING SYSTEM

I have tried to explain the action of breathing and its interaction with the blood circulation, because unless we realize something of the mechanism which is working, some very odd ideas can arise.[23] Some people say 'breathing and oxygen is so important – let's have as much of it as we can', and they try to flood their blood stream with oxygen by long deep breaths or by holding the breath. We must not forget that the breathing centres in the low brain – below consciousness – are there to monitor what is happening and to keep the balance of oxygen and carbon dioxide required by our activity by regulating the kind of breathing we do.

So if you suddenly decide, as you lie motionless on the floor, to do some deep breathing or to take a deep breath and hold it in the hope of 'taking in more oxygen', all you achieve is to muddle up all this finely tuned and balanced control, and you may get a feeling of dizziness too. You may be told this does not matter or even that it is doing you good by 'flooding your brain with oxygen' or 'inducing relaxation'. In fact, what you are inducing is total unconsciousness as the breathing centres are swamped by oxygen which they cannot use, and as you wash out from the blood in the lungs more and more carbon dioxide which would otherwise act as a regulator of breathing. I suppose the breathing centres hope that if you become unconscious you will stop being so silly as to try to take over their job, which they know better than you; and they can then carry on.

In the same way, if a child holds his breath to frighten and bully you into doing his will, you need not worry. The breathing centres will cause him to start breathing again, as the carbon dioxide content of the blood rises, because it is not being interchanged in the lungs. It is said that the breath can only be held for forty seconds before control is re-established.[24] In this way, as so often happens, the wisdom of the body confounds our own wilful silliness, and prevents us from damaging ourselves beyond repair.

If you remember that the carbon dioxide is manufactured and the oxygen used up by *working* muscles, then you are obviously upsetting the plan if you attempt to do deep breathing while the body is lying at rest. It is just like sitting in a car and forcing your foot down on the accelerator pedal while the gear is still in neutral.

If one asks someone to 'take a deep breath' the tendency is for them to begin by sucking in the air noisily through the mouth or by sniffing it in equally noisily through the nose, then to lift the chest and breathe high in front, or else push out the abdomen. Both these movements are performed by extension of the spine, the first tilting the whole chest up towards the chin but not expanding it in any way, the second simply stretching the abdominal muscles, which is no help to the chest. The only way to expand the chest in its three dimensions, and so really to breathe deeply, is by a true movement of the diaphragm, plus rib movement.

It is an excellent thing to 'lift up the chest' and 'hold the head high' but these should be recognized as upper spinal movements and performed with care. They in no way help the *expansion* of the chest in its three dimensions which is what is wanted for deep breathing. They just lift the whole chest into a better position so that expansion can then more comfortably take place.

In some people the action of the diaphragm is very weak and has to be encouraged. This is sometimes done by teaching them to let the abdominal wall come gently forwards as they breathe in, and fall back equally gently, when breathing out.[25] Nothing should be forced or other muscles are used, for example back muscles. Some people imagine the diaphragm is the upper part of the abdomen and that it goes inwards and outwards as they breathe. They usually have rather a narrowed lower chest with practically no movement, perhaps 1 inch (2·5 cms) expansion instead of the normal $3\frac{1}{2}-4\frac{1}{2}$ ins (8·7–10 cms). Other people have to be taught to use the lower rib movement. Both these types have the habit of quick upper chest breathing which can lead to hyperventilation. This means getting rid of too much carbon dioxide and thus upsetting the breathing centres. It can also be associated with anxiety states and other difficulties.

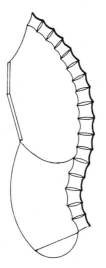 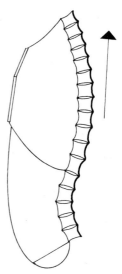

Cramping of the
upper spine, chest,
and abdomen

Upward and backward movement of the
upper spine gives ample chest room and
relieves weight on abdomen

A properly balanced movement of diaphragm and ribs is the ideal, and should always be incorporated with any other training. This is done by allowing no lower abdominal protrusion and only slight bulging between the rib angles in front, coupled with sideways and upwards movement of the lower ribs. This can easily be achieved by placing the hands on the lower ribs, and finger-tips between the angle in front. Feel gentle movement as described above as you breathe in. Breathe out easily and feel the ribs fall down again.[26]

Bearing all this in mind, the wise thing to do is gradually to increase your need for, and use of, oxygen by carefully selected exercise, i.e. aerobic training. As you put your muscles to work, they will use more oxygen and produce more carbon dioxide which immediately will stimulate your breathing centres.[27]

KEEPING THE BLOOD FLOWING

Muscular activity, movement, and exercise, is absolutely essential to preserve and increase not merely breathing but your blood circulation too.[28] The playing arm of any professional tennis player is a living example of this relationship. Its bones will be thicker and stronger than the bones in the other arm because the extra work it does brings in more blood and therefore more bone salts.

Anything up to 75 per cent of the four to six litres of blood that the body contains can be concentrated on active muscles. This is part of the fundamental principle lying behind aerobic training, the other part being the increased blood supply to the lungs. Other areas therefore get less. This is the reason for not eating a heavy meal before exercise, as the digestive system will not be receiving enough blood to get on with its work, and you may feel ill.

Another aspect of circulation which must be touched on concerns the veins of the legs. There are pockets (valves) attached to the inside walls of these veins in pairs with their open ends upwards. This means that as the blood flows along quickly its force closes the pockets; but if the flow gets really slow, the blood will fill the pockets, which will bulge open and so prevent it flowing backwards. Blood easily pools in the legs and abdominal veins as they are furthest away from the thrust of the heart beat. This is why all foot and ankle movements are particularly useful since they cause the muscles to pump the blood up the legs against the force of gravity and so back to the heart. Diaphragmatic contraction also helps.

THE NOSE

Normal breathing takes place through the nose.[29] This is very important because the inside of the nose and the breathing passages are especially equipped to heat, dampen, and clean the air before it enters our lungs. Inside the nose, as well as the organs of smell, there are on either side very fine bony layers with a lot of blood in them. These act like little radiators and warm the blood as it flows over them. The air is also lightly bounced about in these irregular damp warm passages so that pieces of dirt can be shaken out. These then fall on the damp mucous surface where they are trapped. There are also tiny hairs (cilia) protruding through the damp mucus. These have a wave-like rhythmic movement which drives the particles and mucus on towards the throat where they can be swallowed. The windpipe (trachea) and upper breathing passages (bronchi) are also lined with the mucus-making cells and with the cells carrying cilia. The body takes special care to keep strange matter and extra fluid out of the lungs. In prolonged or strenuous exercise, the need for interchange of oxygen and carbon dioxide is so great, that we also breathe through our mouths. As soon as is convenient, nose breathing should be resumed, and should always be actively encouraged by all teachers of movement when possible.

5. Exercises sitting on a stool

'The East has recognised long ago that that which is good for man – for his body and for his soul – must also be agreeable, even though at the beginning some resistance must be overcome.'
Erich Fromm, *The Art of Loving*

The movement schemes in this chapter and the next form a safe, comprehensive system of exercise for the whole body aimed at encouraging natural, graceful posture and movement in your everyday life. The selected movements will carefully loosen your joints to their full normal range and strengthen your muscles sufficiently for everyday use without overdeveloping them. You should also develop an awareness of your own body posture and be able to correct it at will.

Some points to remember throughout Chapters 5 and 6:

1) Read each exercise through carefully before doing it for the first time, particularly the 'Cautions'. There is no need to read the last section headed 'Main Muscle Groups', however, unless you have a particular interest in this.

2) Add the 'Repetitions' and progressions mentioned with the exercises as you feel you can accomplish them with ease. Never force or overstrain in any exercise; it can only do you harm. The way to progress is always gently and carefully as you feel your body can adapt to a little more work.

3) Remember you will feel the movements that you do, in your joints. You cannot feel muscles, although you may feel the pull on skin which is very sensitive.

4) When you practise the exercises, try to concentrate fully on what you are doing and enjoy it. You need only repeat a movement a very few times if you do it with your whole attention and with an understanding of what you are trying to achieve. This is why we have put at the beginning of each exercise 'What it's for'. For a fuller understanding of the purpose of the exercises, the theory in the preceding chapters is invaluable.

5) Whatever exercise you are doing, try to maintain the Corrected Posture that applies to the exercise at the same time. Remember, the exercises are not a chore to be got through and then forgotten about, but a means of training your body awareness and posture awareness so that you have better posture and freedom of movement.

6) Breathing instructions are given with most of the exercises. If you find these confusing, just breathe normally. Breathe in and out through the nose whenever possible.

7) Hands. In a number of the exercises that follow you will be asked to clasp your hands. This is always done in the same way, whether the hands are in front of you or behind. Try it first with the hands in front so that you can see what you are doing.

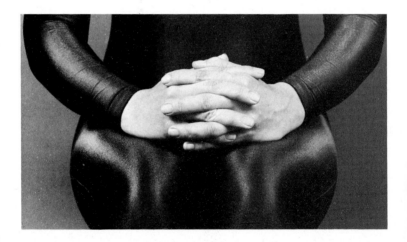

Put your hands in your lap, palms facing the body, little fingers touching thighs. Slide the fingers along the backs of the hands until they interlock. Probably, you will discover that each time you interlock the fingers you tend to put the same forefinger on top, so the same little finger is touching your thigh. It is just a matter of habit. It is a good idea to change the grip halfway through an exercise and put the other forefinger on top instead, so that you do not favour one side of the body. The same applies when you clasp the hands behind you. Take the hands to the back of the body, slide the fingers along the backs of the hands with the palms facing upwards. Feel which forefinger is closest to the back of the body, then change the grip so that the other forefinger touches the body. *Caution.* Do not clench the hands tightly together, rather slide them loosely into position without tension.

8) A check list of small but significant adjustments to run through both when doing exercises and throughout your day.

Eyes soft, not staring.
If you find you are holding your breath, breathe out easily.
Lips soft and lightly closed, not pursed.
Teeth not clenched together, a little space between the top and lower teeth.
Tongue at ease in the mouth, not clamped tightly to the roof of the mouth.
Do a three-point pull whenever you remember (see p. 70).
Try not to sag in the middle of the body.
Do not arch your back, however slightly; stretch and lengthen it upwards.

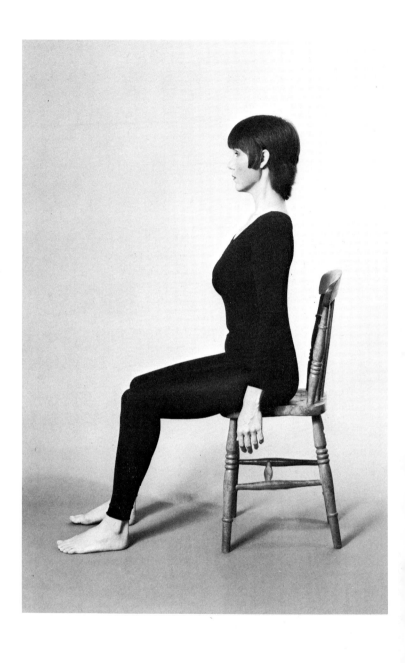

Corrected sitting position

This is the starting position for the first twenty-two exercises. Sit on a hard chair or stool.

Feet. The feet are resting on the floor, hip-width apart and pointing very slightly outwards.

Knees. The knees are bent comfortably, at about a right angle.

Thighs. The thighs are hip-width apart.

Pelvis. You control the tilt of the pelvis, as in standing (see p. 70).

Ribs. Lift the ribcage up away from the hips by stretching your upper back, so there is length in the centre of the body. Do not keep the abdomen pulled in tightly.

Shoulders. The shoulders are down away from the ears.

Neck. The back of the neck is lengthened upwards.

Head. The chin is held at about a right angle to the front of the neck, ears directly above the shoulders.

Neck exercises

This exercise programme starts off by stretching and strengthening the muscles of the neck, and the shoulder area. It is very important to work on these two areas first because any tendency to tenseness and tightness there will increase as you work other areas of the body. The neck and shoulders always have priority, so if you find you are straining them in order to do something in another part of the body, beware. That exercise is probably too hard for you and will not do you good.

1. Head tilting forwards
2. Head pressing backwards
3. Head tilting sideways
4. Head tilting diagonally forwards

SPECIAL USES

1. It is very helpful to do the neck exercises two or three times throughout the day to try to prevent tension in the neck and shoulders building up. Without including the arms, you can press the chin in and tilt the head in the various directions given to stretch the neck at any time.

2. Migraine sufferers often find these exercises very effective in helping to relieve their complaint. However, it is important to practise the exercises regularly, preferably for about a couple of minutes three times a day, rather than remembering to do them just when a headache is coming on. Then it is usually too late.

3. These exercises can also be very helpful in coping with pre-menstrual tension.

CAUTIONS

Never pull or jerk the neck. It is delicate. Work gently and be very mindful of what you are doing. Do not be alarmed if you feel quite strong stretches at first, but progress cautiously. If the stretch is too severe for you when you begin, do the exercise without using the arms at all, gradually progressing over a period of weeks or even months to the full positions. Then add the arms and start again from the beginning and gradually progress as before.

The seven joints of the neck are always being compressed by the heavy weight of the head on top of them, so it is dangerous to circle the head around in one continuous movement. This may damage the delicate joints by grinding them together under such a heavy weight.

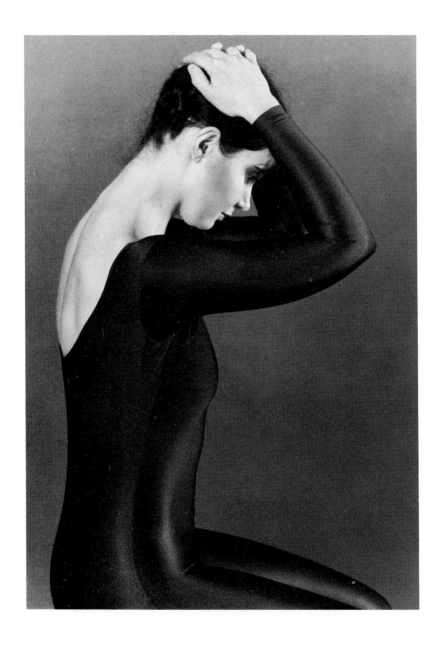

1. *Head tilting forwards*

What it's for. Stretching and strengthening the straight muscles of the neck and upper back.

Starting position. Corrected Sitting. Clasp the hands loosely on the upper part of the back of the skull where they act as extra weight. Have the elbows forwards at either side of the face just above eye level. No undue tension in the arms or shoulders. Press the chin inwards and retain this throughout the exercise.

What you do and what you feel
1. Carefully tilt the head forward, keeping the chin in, until you feel a stretch in the back of the neck. Do not push with the arms.
2. Try to hold the position until the stretching at the back of the neck subsides, but lift the head a little if the stretch becomes too much.
3. Tilt the head further forwards if you feel you can take a bit more stretch.
4. Gently lift the head and lower the arms.

Repetitions and how to progress. If you do not feel very much stretch in the back of the neck, make the arms heavier by bringing the elbows closer together and loosening the clasped hands a little. If the stretch subsides, do a Pelvic Tilt as on page 127, while the head pulls downwards. Go on stretching the neck and back in this way until it feels loosened. Then slowly lift the head and lower the arms.

Breathing. IN at the start, OUT as the head goes forward. Breathe normally as you hold your position.

Main muscle groups
Flexors and Extensors of the head and neck.
Retractors of the chin.

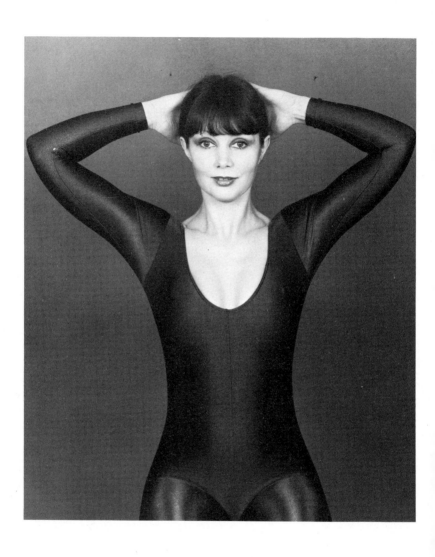

2. *Head pressing backwards*

What it's for. Strengthening the muscles at the back of the neck by static muscle work. See page 34.

Starting position. Corrected Sitting. Clasp the hands loosely on the back of the head. Press the chin inwards and retain this throughout the exercise.

What you do and what you feel
1. Press the head backwards into the hands, pressing forwards with the hands at the same time, so the head does not actually move.
2. Stop, holding the head and hands in position. Press again and stop.

Repetitions and how to progress. Repeat mindfully two to six times as you feel able.

Breathing. IN with the starting position, OUT as you press the head backwards against the resisting hands.

Caution. Never overdo neck work. If you find this exercise difficult, try it lying on the floor so the head is supported, and press the head into the floor (no arms).

Main muscle groups
Extensors of head and neck.
Retractors of chin.

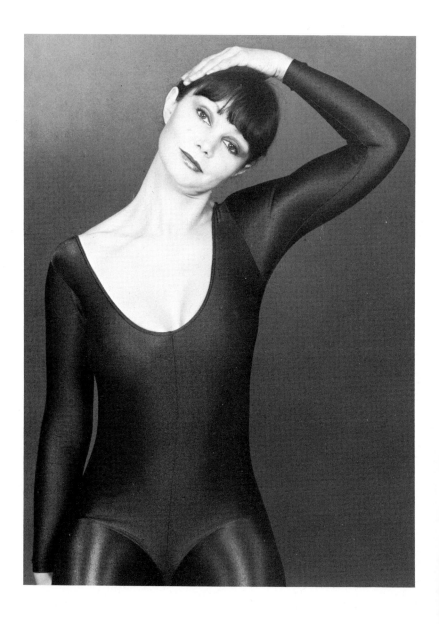

3. *Head tilting sideways*

What it's for. Stretches and strengthens the muscles at the sides of the neck.

Starting position. Corrected Sitting. Place the left hand across the top of the head to act as extra weight. Press the chin inwards and keep it there.

What you do and what you feel
1. Tilt the head sideways to the left until you feel a stretch in the right side of the neck. Do not push the head with the hand. Keep the right shoulder well pulled down by lightly holding onto the leg of the chair with your right hand.
2. Hold the position where you feel a good, but bearable stretch, keeping the chin in.
3. Lift the head a little if the stretch becomes too much and then tilt it further if you feel you can take a bit more.
4. Lift the head upright and lower the arm.
5. Do the exercise to the right using the right arm.

There is no need to repeat the side-stretching of the neck more than once on each side.

Breathing. IN at the start, OUT as the head tilts sideways. Breathe normally as you hold the side-stretch position.

Cautions. See page 86.

Main muscle groups
Retractors of chin.
Side Flexors of head.

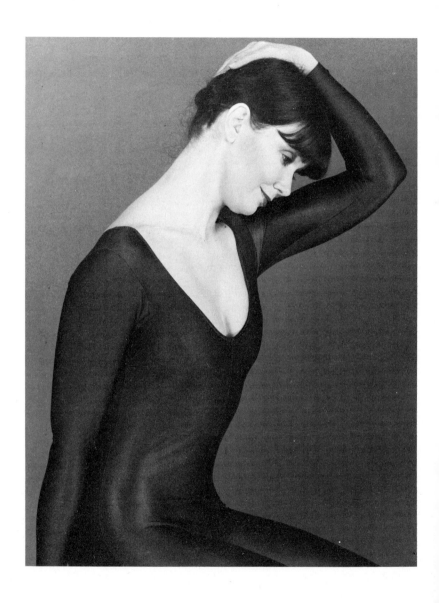

4. *Head tilting diagonally forwards*

What it's for. Stretches and strengthens the diagonal muscles of the neck and upper back.

Starting position. Corrected Sitting. Face squarely toward one wall of the room. Turn the head only (not the shoulders) a quarter turn to face the left front corner of the room. Put the left hand across the top of the head so that the finger-tips touch the right side of the back of the skull behind the ear. Hold the stool with the right hand to anchor the right arm. Press the chin inwards and keep it there.

What you do and what you feel
1. Tilt the head forwards so that your forehead faces down towards your left knee. You should feel a stretch from the right shoulder blade to the base of the skull on the right.
2. Hold the position where you feel a good but bearable stretch, keeping the chin in.
3. Lift the head upright and lower the arm.
4. Now do the exercise facing the right front corner of the room using the right arm.

Breathing. IN at the start, OUT as the head tilts diagonally forwards. Breathe normally as you hold the position.

Caution. See page 86.

Main muscle groups
Retractors of chin.
Rotators, Flexors and Extensors of head.

Shoulder girdle exercises

We all tend to allow our shoulder girdles to drop forwards. It is a continuous battle to keep them back in place and down away from the ears, so that the chest is lifted, the ribcage and the abdominal area not squeezed and the back not rounded (see p. 165). These exercises help tremendously in this battle and also tend to relieve aches and pains and tightness at the top of the back. The shoulder girdle is composed of the shoulder blade and collar bone (scapula and clavicle – see skeleton pic. p. 48).

5. Shoulder lift and squeeze
6. Shoulder-blade squeeze
7. Upper arm backward squeeze
8. Advanced shoulder girdles exercise

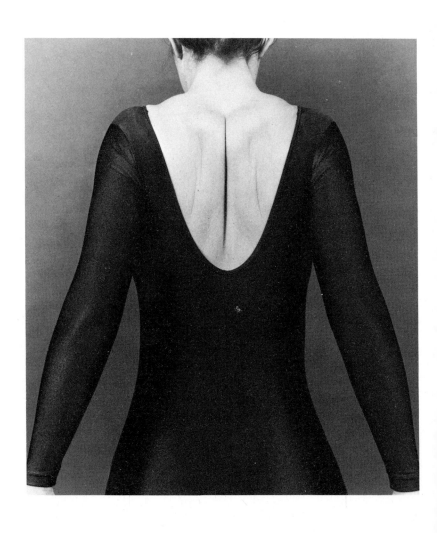

5. *Shoulder lift and squeeze*

What it's for. Contracts the muscles at the top of the back to counteract the forward pull by gravity on the shoulder girdles. It is a good warming-up exercise before doing stronger exercises which include the weight of the arms.

Starting position. Corrected Sitting.

What you do and what you feel
1. Lift the shoulder girdles up as near to the ears as you can get them.
2. Pull the shoulder girdles back as far as you can, keeping them up as high as possible.
3. Return to the Starting Position with a three-point pull (see p. 70).

Repetitions and how to progress. Repeat movements 1, 2 and 3 four times at first. Gradually work up to about six repetitions. Progress to pulling the head back so you look at ceiling with movement 2, lift the head as you do movement 3.

Breathing. IN with movement 1, OUT with movements 2 and 3.

Cautions. Try not to involve the arms unnecessarily in the exercise; just keep them hanging at your sides. Try to make the shoulder girdles do all the work as this uses the selected muscles.

Main muscle groups
Trapezius, ant. and post. folds of Axilla, outward Rotators of shoulder joints.
Elevators and Retractors of shoulder girdles.
Extensors of head.

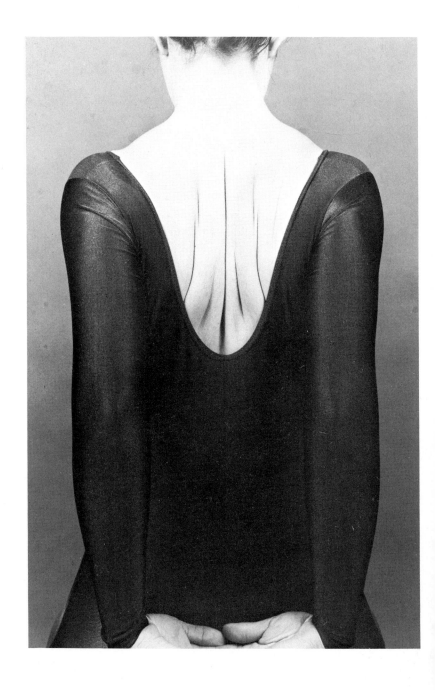

6. Shoulder-blade squeeze

What it's for. Strengthens the muscles which pull the shoulder blades together and pull back the arms. At the same time this exercise lifts the ribcage so that it is in a better position for movement of the lower ribs in breathing.

Starting position. Corrected Sitting. Clasp hands loosely behind the back with the elbows slightly bent.

What you do and what you feel
1. Draw the shoulder blades together and at the same time, press the upper arms towards each other across the back. Do not straighten the elbows.
2. Rest, keeping the hands in position.

Repetitions and how to progress. Repeat three times at first and then progress to about six mindful repetitions.

Breathing. IN with movement 1, OUT with movement 2.

Caution. Do not arch the back.

Main muscle groups
Retractors of shoulder girdles.
Extensors of shoulder joints.

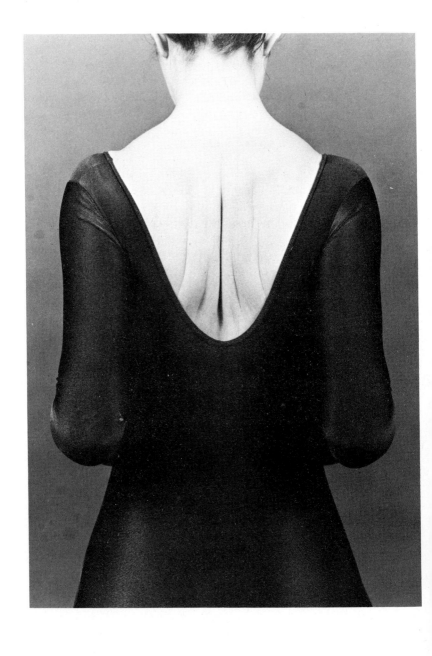

7. Upper arm backwards squeeze

What it's for. Tightens the diagonal muscles crossing the back, which are vital for good posture.

Starting position. Corrected Sitting. Place the palms of the hands flat on the lower ribs in front of the body.

What you do and what you feel. Pull elbows back towards the spine in short jerks. Feel the upper arms pressing backwards strongly. Allow the hands to move slightly as the elbows pull back.

Repetitions. Repeat several times making the movement short, sharp and strong.

Breathing. IN with the starting postion, OUT as you press the elbows back.

Cautions. Try not to tense the front of the neck or raise the shoulders. If your upper arms are very long or your torso very narrow, guard against your elbows banging together.

Main muscle groups
Extensors of shoulder joints.

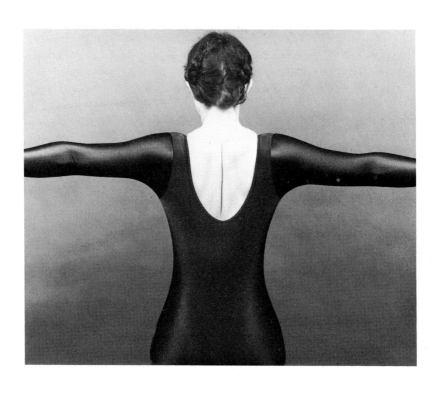

8. *Advanced shoulder girdles exercise*

What it's for. This is a strong exercise for the shoulder girdles. It strengthens the muscles of the upper back. At the same time it lifts the chest in front.

Starting position. Corrected Sitting. Lift the arms out sideways to shoulder level and stretch the finger-tips as far away from the centre of the body as possible, making space across the upper chest. Make a loose fist with the fingers.

What you do and what you feel
1. Pull the shoulder blades together and hold them there.
2. Pull the arms backwards in short jerks one to four times (letting the arms move slightly forwards between each backward pull). Make sure the arms remain at shoulder level.

Repetitions and how to progress. Gradually increase from four to twelve backward pulls.

Cautions. This exercise works the muscles controlling the shoulder girdles more strongly than the previous ones because it includes the weight of the arms. It should be attempted only when the previous shoulder girdle exercises have been mastered. Do not allow the lower back to arch as you press the arms back.

Main muscle groups
Abductors of shoulder joints.
Retractors of shoulder girdles.
Extensors of shoulder joints.

Arms, breasts and hands exercises

These help prevent stiffness in the shoulder, elbow, wrist, and finger joints. They also tighten up the contours of the arms, and help to lift the breasts.

  9. Pressing arms back and rotation inwards
10. Rotating the arms outwards and inwards
11. Advanced rotation of the arms
12. Breast-lifting exercise
13. Hand-stretching exercise

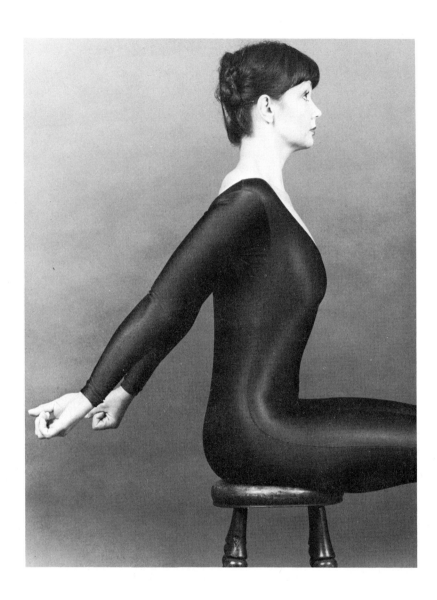

9. *Pressing arms back and rotation inwards*

What it's for. Tightens up the back of the upper arm, a part that so many women complain has 'gone to flab'. Encourages inward rotation of the lower arms and shoulder joints, so necessary for putting the arms into a jacket. Strengthens muscles across the back.

Starting position. Corrected Sitting. Hands loosely fisted.

What you do and what you feel
1. Bend the elbows fully (so that your fists come up to your shoulders in front of you), turning the fingers to face the shoulders. Keep your elbows near your ribcage.
2. Straighten the elbows very quickly, turning the arms inwards and pressing them behind you in one strong movement (see illustration opposite).

Repetitions and how to progress. Repeat movements 1 and 2 four times at first and progress to eight and then twelve repetitions.

Breathing. IN with movement 1, OUT with movement 2.

Cautions. Do not be surprised if the backs of the upper arms feel a little stiff for a day or two after you have done the exercise. It is a strong exercise but very effective.

Main muscle groups
Flexors of the elbow joints.
Extensors of the elbow joints.
Medial Rotators of shoulder joints.
Supinators and Pronators of forearm.

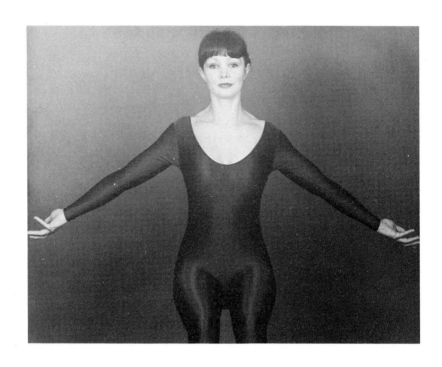

10. *Rotating the arms outwards and inwards*

What it's for. Rotation of the shoulder joints and lower arms in order to prevent stiffness.

Starting position. Corrected Sitting.

What you do and what you feel
1. Lift the elbows slightly and turn the hands outwards fully, straightening the elbows (see illustration opposite).
2. Slightly bend the elbows and turn the hands inwards fully, then restraighten the elbows.

Repetitions. As often as you like.

Cautions. The rotation in the forearms and shoulder joints should be a flowing movement. Remember to keep the shoulders down away from the ears throughout.

Main muscle groups
Abductors of shoulder joints.
Medial and lateral Rotators of shoulder joints.
Pronators and Supinators of forearms.

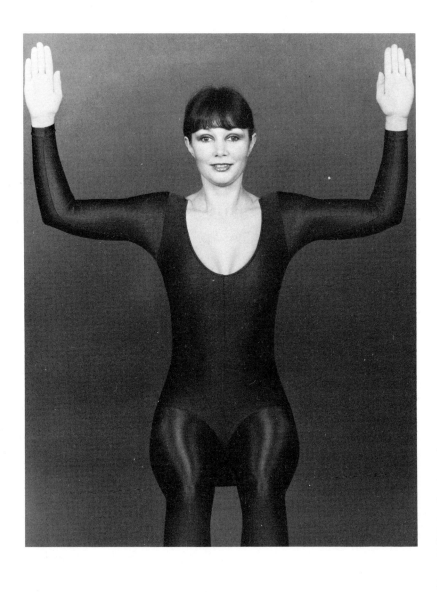

11. *Advanced rotation of the arms*

What it's for. Strengthening the muscles in the shoulder joints that rotate the arms.

Starting position. Corrected Sitting. Arms out sideways at shoulder level. Raise the lower arms to form right angles at the elbows, keeping the upper arms at shoulder level (see illustration opposite).

What you do and what you feel
1. Push the lower arms downwards and then as far back as possible without letting the shoulder girdles or elbows move.
2. Raise the lower arms to right angles again and press backwards.

Repetitions. As often as you like.

Breathing. OUT with movement 1, IN with movement 2.

Cautions. Keep the shoulders down away from the ears and maintain a right angle at the elbows throughout the exercise.

Main muscle groups
Abductors of shoulder joints.
Medial and lateral Rotators of shoulder joints.

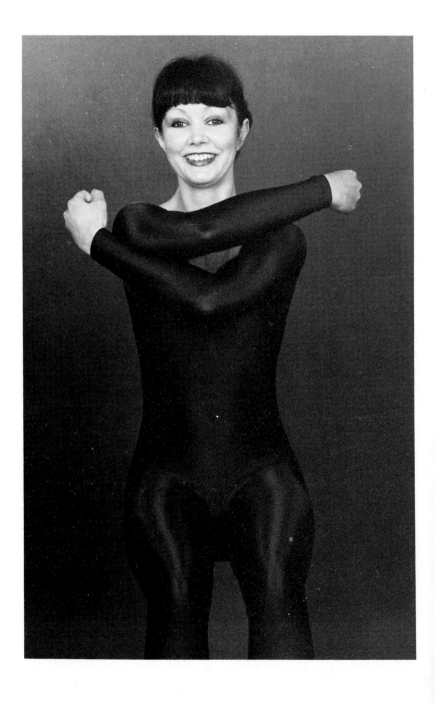

12. *Breast-lifting exercise*

What it's for. Strengthening the muscles which lie behind the breasts and help to support them.

Starting position. Corrected Sitting. Arms out sideways at shoulder level, elbows straight, palms facing front, make loose fists with the hands.

What you do and what you feel
1. Bring the arms upwards strongly so they cross over in front of your face, elbows bending slightly. Press further across.
2. Return to the starting position.
3. Repeat with the opposite arm on top in the crossed-over position.
4. Repeat with arms crossing at shoulder level.
5. Repeat with arms crossing at breast level.

Repetitions and how to progress. Work up to four repetitions of movements 1, 2 and 3 at each level.

Breathing. IN with the starting position, OUT with the cross-over movement.

Caution. Keep the shoulders well down away from the ears.

Main muscle groups
Abductors of shoulder joints.
Flexors of shoulder joints especially Pectoralis Major.
Extensors of shoulder joints.
Flexors and Extensors of elbow joints.

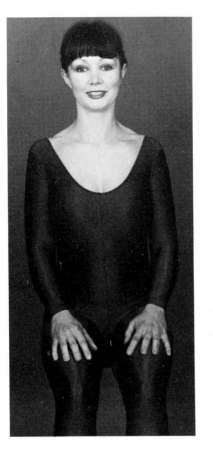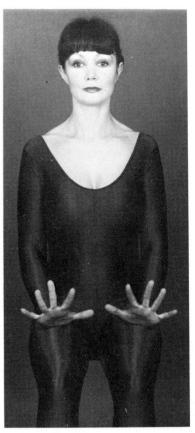

13. *Hand-stretching exercise*

What it's for. Stretching the fingers and thumbs to prevent stiffness.

Starting position. Corrected Sitting. Place the hands on the thighs, palms down.

What you do and what you feel
1. Lift the hands up and stretch out and open the fingers and thumbs as much as possible.
2. Let the hands drop back onto the thighs.
3. Repeat several times.

Cautions. Keep the wrists resting on your thighs and do not lift the shoulders.

Main muscle groups
Extensors of wrists.
Extensors of fingers and thumbs.
Abductors of fingers and thumbs.

Abdominal and back exercises

Exercises 14–17 are to shorten and tighten up the abdominal muscles in all directions. They also work the complementary muscles of the back. See Chapter 3 pp. 56, 57, 59, 60.

14. Waist side bends
15. Waist twist
16. Waist diagonal bend
17. The pelvic tilt

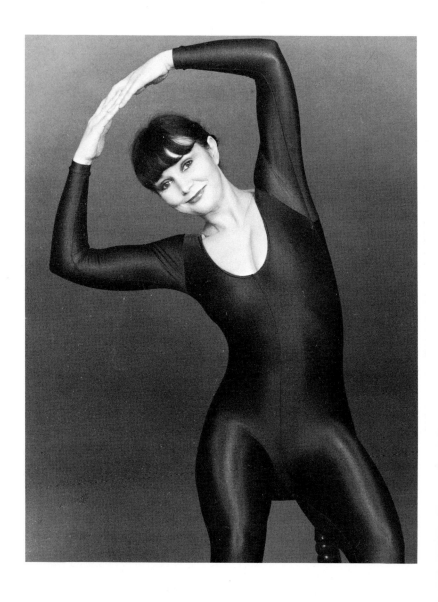

14. *Waist side bends*

What it's for. Stretches and strengthens the muscles at the side of the trunk, back and front (see pp. 56–60). This is a very good example of fully stretching and then fully contracting a group of muscles (see p. 37). Mobilizes the five joints of the lower back.

Starting position. Corrected Sitting. Clasp the hands just above the head. Elbows out sideways. Do a three-point pull (p. 70).

What you do and what you feel
1. Bend sideways to the right as far as you can, keeping the pelvis firmly on the chair. Hold the position for a few seconds.
2. Come up a little then try to bend further. Do this three or four times.
3. Come up to the starting position. Repeat to the other side.

Repetitions and how to progress. Repeat this sequence twice. Work up to about four repetitions.

Breathing. IN with the starting position, OUT as you bend sideways. Breathe normally as you do the small further bends.

Cautions. Do not allow the chest to sag or rotate. If it is too tiring for you to keep your arms above your head for the exercise, place them on your upper chest instead, as in the next exercise.

Main muscle groups
Side Flexors of trunk (abdominal and back muscles).

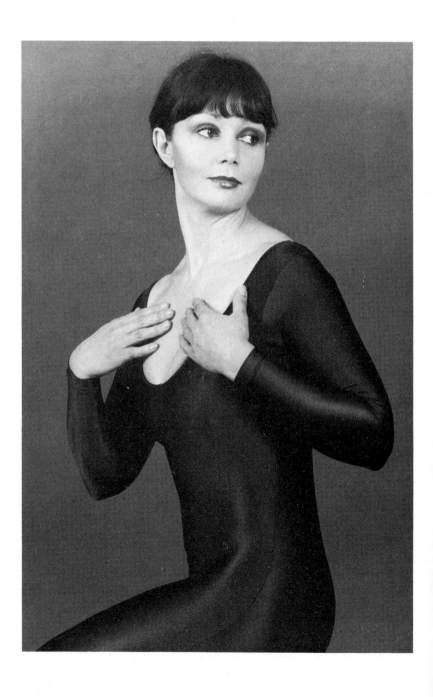

15. *Waist twist*

What it's for. The diagonal muscles of the abdomen, back and neck. Mobilizes the joints of the upper back and neck.

Starting position. Corrected Sitting. Place the hands flat on the upper chest.

What you do and what you feel
1. Lift the ribcage up away from the hips, creating space in the centre of the body.
2. Keep the lift and twist round to the left, turning your head and looking round as far as you can. The pelvis must remain facing forwards.
3. Go on pressing round in small further movements, with the head and upper body.
4. Face front again. Repeat to the other side.

Repetitions and how to progress. Increase the number of small further movements on each side.

Breathing. IN with the first movement, OUT as you twist. Breathe normally as you do the small further twists.

Caution. Try not to lift the shoulders.

Main muscle groups
Rotators of head, neck and trunk (abdominal, back and neck muscles).

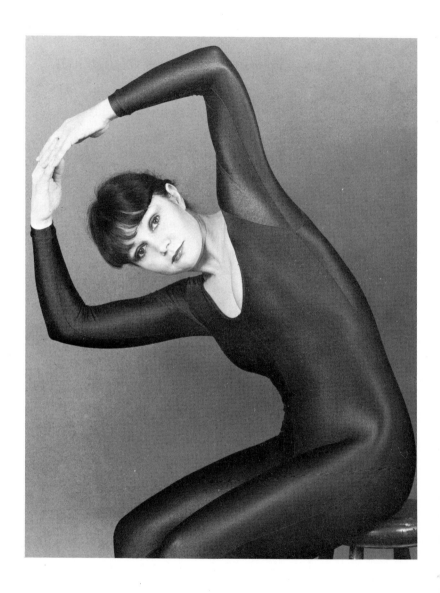

16. *Waist diagonal bend*

What it's for. Mobilizes the whole spine. Works abdominal and back muscles.

Starting position. Corrected Sitting. Clasp the hands just above the head. Elbows out sideways. Do a three-point pull.

What you do and what you feel
1. Lift ribcage.
2. Twist to the left.
3. Bend towards the right knee as far as you can, keeping the pelvis firmly on the stool.
4. Come up a little, then bend again. Do this three times.
5. Come up fully, retaining the twist. Then turn forwards.
6. Do the sequence on the other side.

Repetitions and how to progress. Increase the number of small further movements on each side.

Breathing. IN as you lift at the start and as you twist to the side. OUT as you bend diagonally downwards. Breathe normally for the small further movements.

Cautions. Do not attempt this exercise if you have any weakness or pain in the lower back as it involves a twist and a bend and it is better to do these movements separately until the back is strong. If it is too tiring for you to keep the arms above the head for the exercise, place them on your upper chest instead.

Main muscle groups
Trunk Rotators.
Trunk Side Flexors.
Back Extensors.

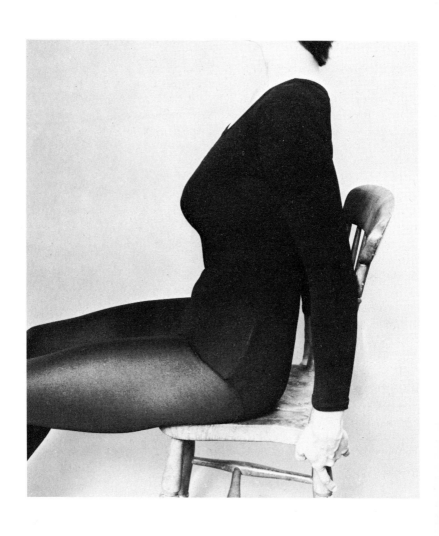

17. *The pelvic tilt*

What it's for. Shortening the straight fibres of the abdominal wall in front (see p. 57). Mobility of the hip joints and lower back. Recognition of movement of the pelvis (see pp. 49, 69–70).

Starting position. Corrected Sitting near the front of the seat. Hands holding the back of the chair seat.

What you do and what you feel
1. Roll the pelvis so that the pubic bone in front comes up towards your nose. The curve of the lower back will straighten and the tummy will be compressed.
2. Return to the starting position.

Repetitions and how to progress. Repeat as often as you like. Try to correct the tilt of the pelvis when standing (see pp. 70, 165).

Breathing. IN with the starting position, OUT as you roll the pelvis backwards.

Caution. Keep upright from the waist.

Main muscle groups
Straight fibres of abdominal muscles in front.

Compare this exercise with the pelvic tilt done in the corrected lying position, p. 153.

Legs and feet exercises

The next set of exercises shapes the contours of the legs and strengthens the feet. Tired feet tend to make you feel tired all over.

At first it may not be pleasant to feel the feet really trying to move when you do the exercises, especially if they are used to being restricted in tight socks or stockings and shoes. However, with practice and concentration the foot exercises become pleasant and can be done whenever you have a moment to spare.

18. Buttocks exercise
19. Kicks
20. Ankle and foot joints exercise
21. Foot exercise
22. Instep exercise

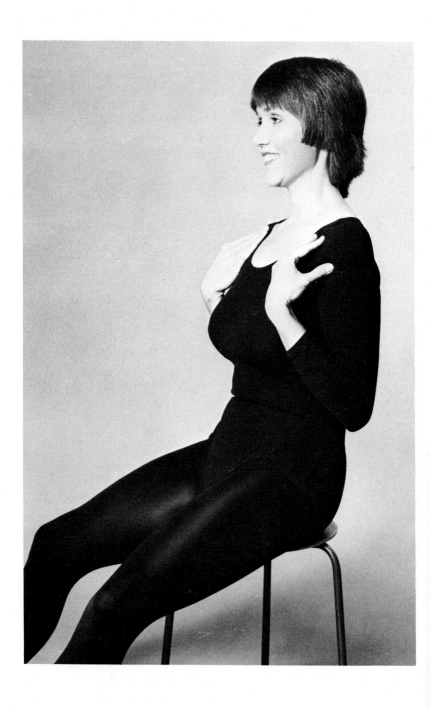

18. *Buttocks exercise*

What it's for. Tightening the buttocks. This exercise is particularly applicable to women, who usually have more fat here than men.

Starting position. Corrected Sitting. Move the feet slightly forwards. Hands resting on the upper chest. Do a Pelvic Tilt (p. 127) and hold it throughout the exercise.

What you do and what you feel
1. Press the thighs downwards and rotate them outwards a little.
2. Stop.

Repetitions and how to progress. Repeat several times. Progress by holding movement 1 longer. Stop when you have had enough. You will know when.

Breathing. IN with starting position, OUT as you do movement 1.

Main muscle groups
Lateral Rotators.
Extensors of hips.

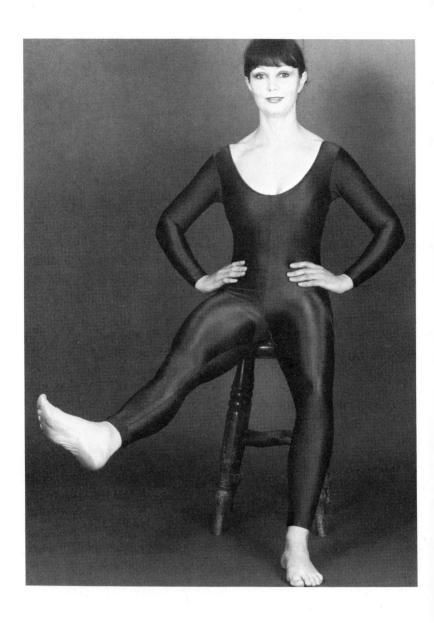

19. *Kicks*

What it's for. Tightens the front of the thighs and increases the circulation.

Starting position. Corrected Sitting. Hands on hips. Do a Pelvic Tilt (p. 127) and turn the thighs outwards. The left foot remains on the floor throughout the exercise. Lift the right leg off the floor a little with the knee slightly bent and the foot bent upwards.

What you do and what you feel
1. Straighten the right leg quickly and sharply, pushing the heel away from you.
2. Return to the starting position.

Repetitions. Repeat the kick several times until the leg begins to tire. Then repeat with the other leg.

Cautions. Be sure to hold the Pelvic Tilt throughout the exercise. Keep the shoulders down away from the ears, and try not to strain the front of the neck as you work. If you have painful knees, leave out this exercise or gently bend and stretch the leg instead of kicking.

Main muscle groups
Lateral Rotators of hip.
Flexors of hip.
Extensors of knee.
Dorsiflexors of ankle.

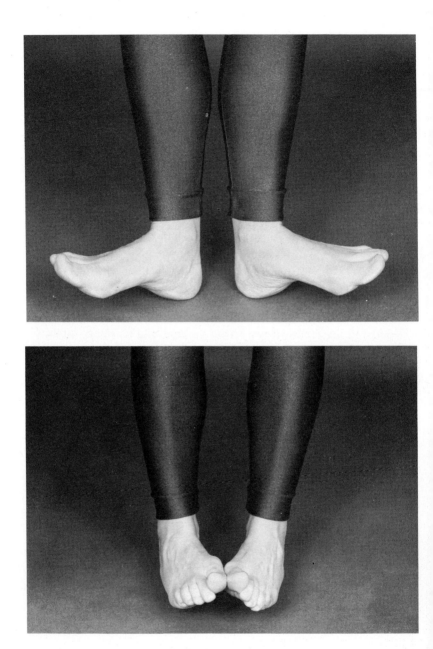

20. *Ankle and foot joints exercise*

What it's for. To strengthen and mobilize the ankles and joints of the feet.

Starting position. Corrected Sitting. Place the feet slightly forwards. Keep the heels on the floor and the knees together throughout the exercise.

What you do and what you feel
1. Brush the feet outwards along the floor, lifting and turning them as much as possible so that the little toes point towards the outside of the calves (see top picture).
2. Drop the feet and brush them inwards along the floor, lifting and turning them as much as possible so that the big toes point towards the inside of the calves (see lower picture).

Repetitions. As often as you like until you begin to tire.

Cautions. Prevent any movement of the knees, so that as much rotation as is possible takes place in the foot joints.

Main muscle groups
Invertors and Evertors of feet.

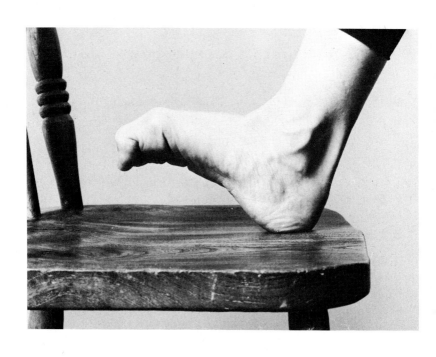

21. *Foot exercise*

What it's for. Mobilizing the small joints of the feet and toes.

Starting position. Corrected sitting. Place the feet slightly forwards. The feet are lifted up towards the shins and the heels are on the floor throughout the exercise.

What you do and what you feel
1. Curl the toes down and in towards the balls of the feet and squeeze tightly. See picture. The foot has been photographed on a chair for clarity.
2. Uncurl the toes and stretch them as much as possible, trying to make space between the toes.

Repetitions. As often as you like, until the feet begin to tire.

Cautions. Be sure that you make the big toes curl under and work as much as possible. Eventually you will be able to see all five bones at the base of the toes pop up as you do movement 1 and lots of space between each toe when you do movement 2.

Main muscle groups
Dorsiflexors of ankle.
Long and short Flexors of toes.
Extensors and Abductors of toes.

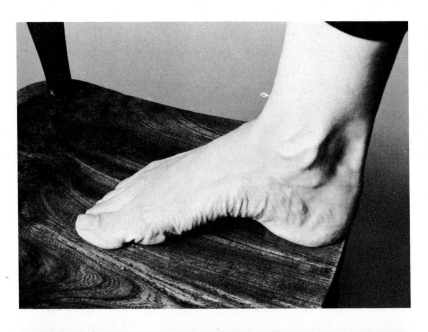

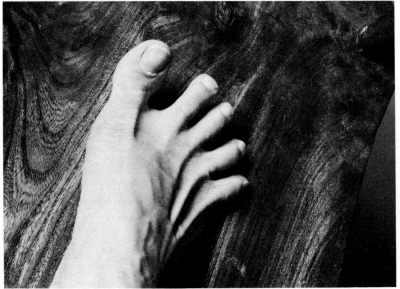

22. *Instep exercise*

What it's for. Strengthening the small muscles of the feet that support the arches.

Starting position. Corrected Sitting. Feet slightly forwards as in the previous exercise.

What you do and what you feel
1. Keep the toes straight and draw them in towards the heels sliding them along the floor, so that you hump up the joints where the toes attach to the feet. See top picture. The foot has been photographed on a chair for clarity.
2. Slide the toes out along the floor again and stretch them, trying to open out the toes.

Repetitions. As often as you like until the feet begin to tire.

Cautions. Do not move the heels and keep the tips of the toes touching the floor.

Main muscle groups
Lumbrical muscles.
Dorsal and Plantar Interossei.

6. Exercises on the floor

'You have considerable choice in the lines your body will assume. Thus you can allow your body, through neglect, to sag, bulge and spread. Or you can so mould your figure as to bring it added grace and vigour.'
Bess M. Mensendieck, *Look Better, Feel Better*

As well as dealing with exercises to be done on the floor for support, this chapter describes what is in effect the final outcome of the whole system – a good standing position. It also gives a brief introduction to the technique of physiological relaxation.

Back control exercises

The next three exercises strengthen the muscles of the back. Unlike the previous exercises, these are performed sitting on the floor. If the first proves difficult for you, be patient, straighten the back for a little while, then let it sag for a bit to give you a rest, and then straighten up again. The same applies to the next two. If I had to choose three vital exercises for someone with very little time to practise, I would choose these three. You gain back control which is essential in your everyday life, you also learn to lift the chest and the abdominal muscles, and you work the arms and legs.

As a teacher, I find these three Back Control Exercises particularly important and useful as safe, testing exercises for the capability of the back to perform work. I find them the best starting point for people with weak backs. Students find it very useful to do them side-ways-on to a mirror, as then they can see the curves of their spines and watch as they gradually correct themselves over a period of time. I encourage students to do them at home as they are very safe and when mastered they usually help enormously with back ache and make a tremendous difference to the rest of their work and their ability to hold a good posture generally (see pp. 66–71).

23. Legs bent
24. Legs apart
25. Legs together

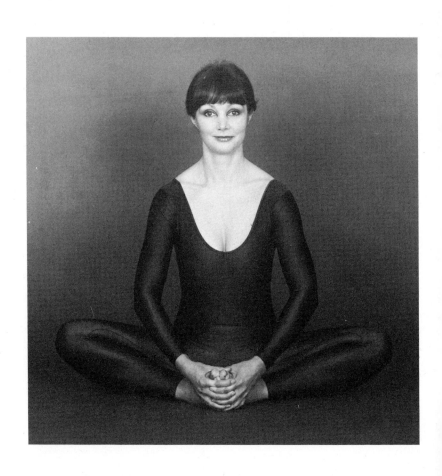

23. *Back control – legs bent*

What it's for
1. Strengthens the back muscles.
2. Mobilizes the hip joints.
3. Stretches the Inward Rotators and Adductors of the hips which tend to shorten and restrict movement.

Starting position. Sitting on the floor with the legs bent, knees dropped outwards and the soles of the feet together. Feet as close to the body as possible. Hands clasped around the toes. If this position feels awkward put a cushion under your bottom and hold the ankles instead of the toes at first.

What you do and what you feel
1. Press the knees towards the floor. Straighten the back, lifting the chest. Do a three-point pull.
2. Hold this position for a short while.

How to progress
1. When you have learnt to hold the back straight sitting upright, lower the trunk slowly forwards keeping the back straight, while gently pressing the knees down further.
2. Hold the position for a few moments.
3. Raise the trunk to the Starting Position.

Breathing. IN with the Starting Position, OUT as you lower the trunk forwards. Breathe normally as you hold the forward position.

Cautions. Keep the chest lifted. It may be some months before you are able to tackle the progression.

Main muscle groups
Extensors of head, back and hips.
Lateral Rotators of hips.

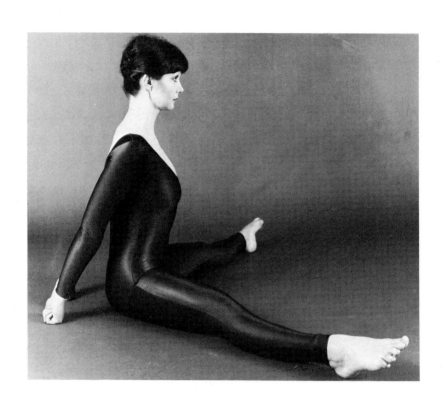

24. *Back control – legs apart*

What it's for
1. Strengthens the back muscles.
2. Mobilizes the hip joints.
3. Stretches the inside thigh muscles (Adductors) which tend to get too short. In this position you will feel slightly more stretch than in Exercise 23.

Starting position. Sit on the floor with the legs as far apart and as straight as is reasonably comfortable. Knee-caps face upwards. Loosely fist the hands and put them on the floor behind you.

What you do and what you feel
1. Push downwards with the hands, straightening the back and lifting the chest. Lift the chest and pull the shoulders down, allowing the elbows to bend a little if necessary.
2. Hold this position for a short time while trying to straighten the knees.
3. Bring the legs together and shake them out along the floor to comfort them.

How to progress
1. As the back muscles get stronger you will no longer need to prop yourself up with the hands, so place them on the inside of the legs at about the knees. Keep the back straight and the chest well lifted. Push with the hands against the inside of the knees if necessary.
2. When Progression 1 becomes easy, then lower the trunk gently forwards, keeping the spine perfectly straight. Hands slide down the legs. Raise the trunk to the starting position.

Cautions. Do not overstretch the insides of the legs. It may be some months before you can tackle the progressions.

Main muscle groups
Extensors of the head, back and shoulder joints.
Retractors of shoulder girdles.
Abductors and Extensors of the hips.
Extensors of knees.

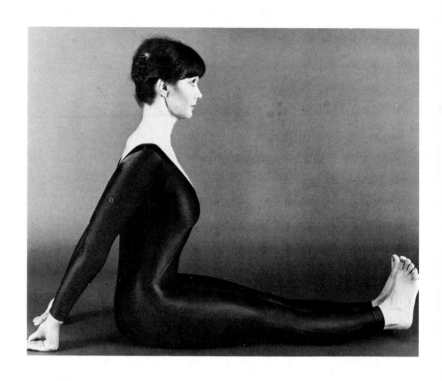

25. *Back control – legs together*

What it's for
1. Strengthens the back muscles.
2. Mobilizes the hip joints.
3. Stretches the muscles on the backs of the thighs and the back of the lower legs.

Starting position. Sit on the floor with the legs straight forwards. The feet are together and pointing upwards towards the face. Knee-caps face upwards. Loosely fist the hands and put them on the floor behind you. If you find this position difficult, put a cushion under your bottom and bend your knees a little.

What you do and what you feel
1. Push downwards with the hands, straightening the back and lifting the chest. Pull the shoulders down and the shoulder blades together, allowing the elbows to bend a little if necessary.
If you have trouble straightening the back, let the legs bend a little.
2. Hold this position for a short time while trying to straighten the knees as much as possible, so that eventually the backs of the knees touch the floor and the heels come off the floor.
3. Take the hands away and try to hold the position for a short time.

(Continued on pp. 148–149)

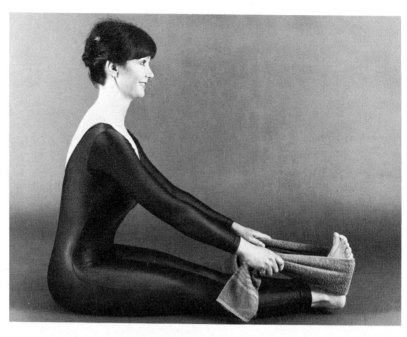

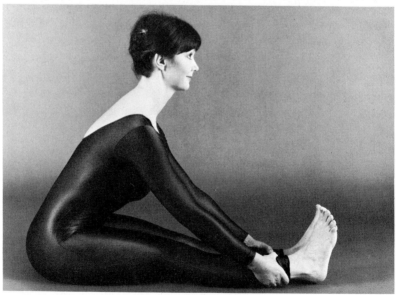

How to progress

1. Place a towel around the middle of the feet and hold it in both hands, palms facing each other. Lift and straighten the torso. Hold this for a short time.

2. When Progression 1 becomes easy, still use the towel and lower the trunk slowly forwards, leading with the front lower ribs. Gradually over a period of some weeks or months hold further and further down the towel, trying to reach the ankles. Make sure the movement forward is from the hips only. The back remains straight and the chest lifted. Hold your position for a short time.

3. Dispense with the towel when you can hold the ankles with your hands. Hold this position for a short time.

4. When you are able, lower the trunk still further, holding the outside edges of the feet.

5. Finally lower the trunk all the way forwards and clasp the hands under the feet. Hold for a short while.

Breathing. IN as you lift the trunk, OUT as you ease it forwards at each stage. Normal breathing as you hold your position.

Cautions. It may take months or even years to achieve the final position. This is not important. What matters most is that you strengthen the postural muscles.

Pregnant women should only go as far as Progression 1.

Main muscle groups

Extensors of head, back and shoulder joints.

Retractors of shoulder girdles.

Extensors of hips, knees and Dorsiflexors of ankles.

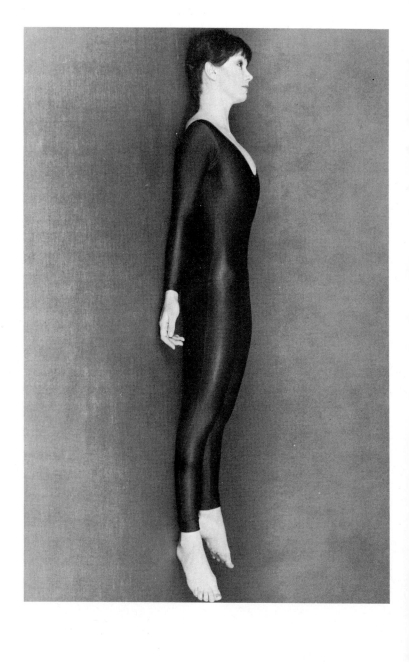

Exercises while lying and kneeling

Corrected lying. Lie flat on your back on the floor, arms at your sides. If you find this painful in the lower back see Cautions below. Bring the feet together. Lift the head and look down the centre of the body to make sure that the breast-bone, navel, crotch and the line between the legs are in a straight line. Replace the head on the floor. Let the feet drop outwards a little. See opposite.

Cautions. If you find that lying flat on the floor causes pain in your lower back, first try placing a thin cushion under your thighs, *not* in the small of the back. If this does not give relief, lie with the knees bent up, feet flat on the floor. Do a Pelvic Tilt (see Exercise 17) and then slowly slide the feet along the floor, letting them turn outwards. You may prefer to slide one leg at a time. Remember to keep the heels in contact with the floor as you straighten the legs, so that their weight is taken by the floor and not by your back. After this, try putting the cushion under your thighs once again if you want it.

26. The pelvic tilt
27. Pelvic side lift
28. Leg-raising sideways
29. Leg-raising backwards
30. The Boat
31. The Ball

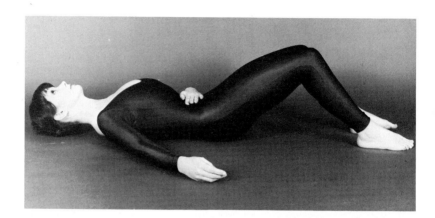

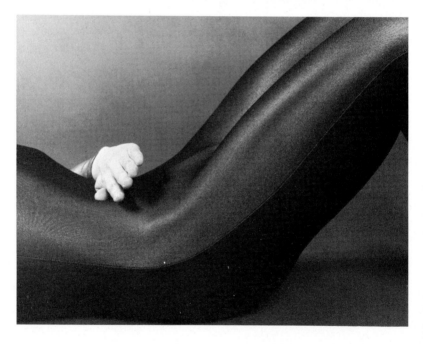

26. *The pelvic tilt*

What it's for. Shortening the straight fibres of the abdominal wall (see p. 57). Mobility of the hip joints and lower back. Recognition of movement of the pelvis in posture control.

Starting position. Corrected Lying. Bend the knees up, keeping the feet flat on the floor, hip-width apart.

What you do and what you feel
1. Roll the pelvis so that the pubic bone in front comes up towards your nose. Your lower back will press onto the floor and your tummy will be compressed.
2. Let the pelvis roll back to the starting position.

Repetitions. Repeat as often as you like.

How to progress
1. Hold the tilted position longer.
2. Do the Pelvic Tilt standing.
3. For women, associate the Pelvic Tilt lying, sitting (p. 127) or standing (pp. 69, 70), with lifting the pelvic floor (see pp. 54, 55).

Breathing. IN with the starting position, OUT as you tilt the pelvis upwards. Breathe normally as you hold the position. Breathe in as the pelvis rolls back to the starting position.

Caution. Keep the shoulders down away from the ears, and the top half of the body quite at ease.

Main muscle groups
Straight fibres of abdominal muscles in front.

Compare this exercise with the pelvic tilt done in the corrected sitting position, p. 127.

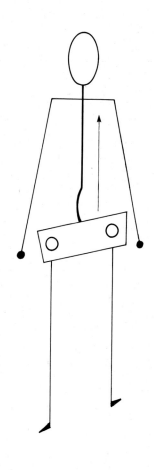

27. *Pelvic side lift*

What it's for. Mobilizing the joints of the lower back (lumbar region). Tightening muscles at the sides of the waist.

Starting position. Corrected Lying.

What you do and what you feel. Lift the right side of the pelvis up towards the ribcage on the right; then push it downwards as you lift up the pelvis on the left.

Repetitions and how to progress. Repeat from side to side as often as you like, slowly and then quickly.

Cautions. Do not lift the hips off the floor as you work. The legs are only moved as a result of the action by the pelvis.

Special Uses. This exercise is particularly helpful for people who tend to get stiff in the lower back, especially after sleep. It can also be done standing, allowing each heel to come off the floor as the pelvis lifts on either side. This is very useful if you have to stand for long periods. Try the exercise standing, starting with the Corrected Standing Position (see p. 165).

Main muscle groups
Side Flexors of trunk.

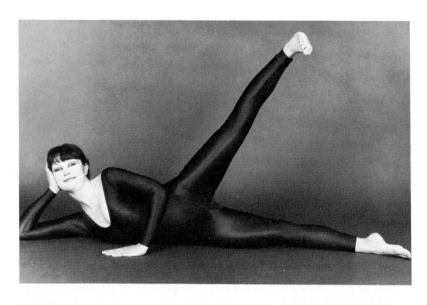

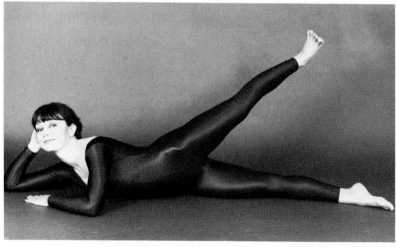

28. *Leg-raising sideways*

What it's for. Very strong training for muscles at the outside of the thighs and the buttocks.

Starting position. Lie on your right side with the body and legs in a straight line. Prop your head up on your right hand. Left-hand palm down on the floor in front of you.

What you do and what you feel

Part 1 (see top picture)
1. Keeping both knees facing forwards, lift the left leg up until the pelvis begins to lift sideways, then hold the position.
2. Lower it to about ten inches off the floor.
3. Repeat movements 1 and 2 as often as you wish.
4. Let the leg rest on the floor.
5. Roll over and repeat the sequence on the other side.

Part 2 (see bottom picture)
1. Lift the left leg up to about 45 degrees.
2. Take it backwards and turn it out, allowing the chest and pelvis to come forwards a little.
3. Lift the leg further up and back as far as possible.
4. Lower the leg to about ten inches off the floor.
5. Repeat movements 3 and 4 as often as you wish.
6. Roll over and repeat the sequence on the other side.

How to progress. Part 1 and 2 of this exercise can also be done standing, starting in the Corrected Standing Position.

Caution. Do not arch or hollow the back.

Main muscle groups
Part 1. Abductors of hips. Extensors of knees. Dorsiflexors of ankles.
Part 2. As above plus Extensors and Outward Rotators of hips. Low Back Extensors.

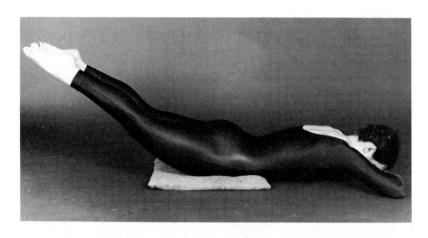

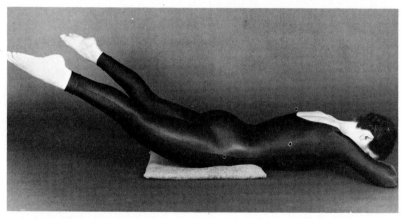

29. *Leg-raising backwards*

What it's for. Tightens up the buttocks and muscles of the outside and inside of the thighs; strengthens the lower part of the long back muscles. This is a very heavy exercise and should only be attempted if you are strong. Do not do it if you have lordosis.

Starting position. Lie on the tummy with a cushion under the pelvis. Bend the elbows and put the hands in front of you on the floor one on top of the other, palms facing down. Rest the forehead on the hands. Do a three-point pull.

What you do and what you feel
Part 1
1. Raise the legs, trying to lift the thighs off the floor. Hold the position for a few moments if you can.
2. Lower the legs gently to the floor and stop.

Part 2
Take the legs apart along the floor. Repeat Part 1.

Repetitions and how to progress
Repeat Parts 1 and 2 up to 8 times as you are able. Progress by raising the legs in Part 2 and then making small circles with the legs at the hip joints, clockwise and then anti-clockwise.

Breathing. Breathe normally. Be sure you do not hold the breath.

Cautions. Work smoothly. If your back is rather weak, lift only one leg at a time and omit the legs apart position until later. If this exercise hurts your back do not do it. First you must strengthen the back with Exercises 23, 24 and 25, sitting on the floor. This exercise is not suitable for pregnant women.

Main muscle groups
Extensors, Abductors and Adductors of hips. Extensors of knees and Plantar Flexors of ankles. Extensors of lower back.

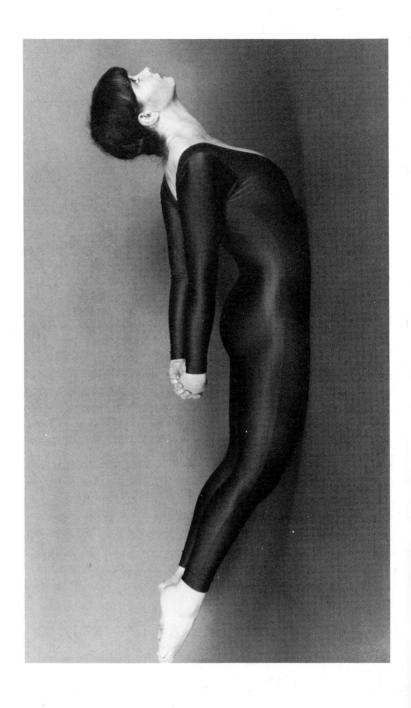

30. *The Boat*

What it's for. Strengthens the long back muscles. Tightens the buttocks, the backs of the thighs and the backs of the arms.

Starting position. Lie on your tummy with your legs together and your feet pointed. Your hands clasped behind you.

What you do and what you feel
1. Lift your chest, arms and legs at the same time and look up. Try to hold the position for a few moments.
2. Lower to the floor.

Repetitions. Not more than four times. You will find it pleasant to follow this exercise with No. 31, The Ball, see next page.

Breathing. IN as you lift, OUT as you lower to the floor.

Cautions. The knees bend very slightly but the main emphasis is on lifting the thighs upwards.
This exercise is unsuitable for pregnant women.

Main muscle groups
Extensors of head, back and hips.
Plantar Flexors of feet and Flexors of toes.
Retractors of shoulder girdles and Extensors of shoulder and elbow joints.

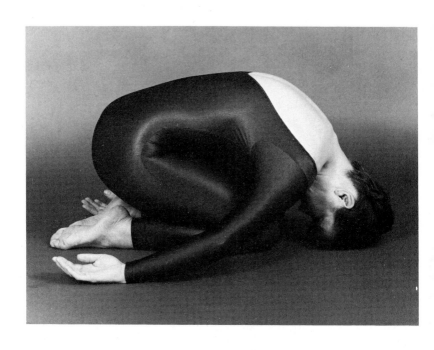

31. *The Ball*

What it's for. Stretching the muscles of the back and neck.

Starting position. Kneeling.

What you do and what you feel
1. Rest your bottom on or near the heels.
2. Curl forwards and tuck your head in towards your knees.
3. Pull your shoulders down and rest the hands, palms up, on the floor on either side.
4. Rest in this position for as long as you please.

Cautions. If you cannot do movement 1 try making a fist with your hands and placing them on the floor behind you, so the arms can take the weight of the body as you gently lower your bottom towards your heels.

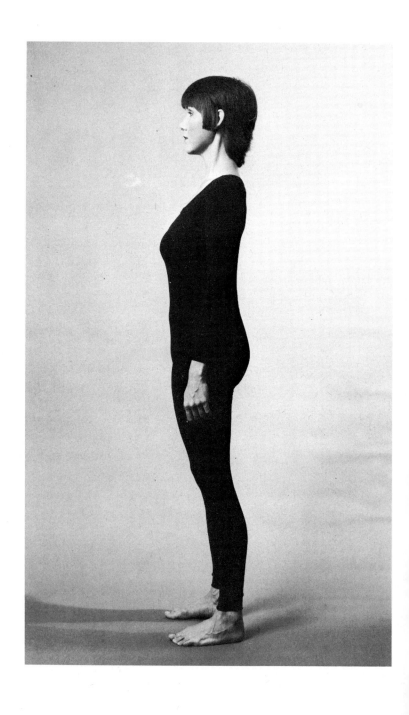

The final aim of all the exercises in Chapters 5 and 6 is that we stand and move about in balance in our daily lives. So let's now consider:

Corrected standing position

Your posture will vary as you move about during the day. Whenever suitable, make the following adjustments which will help you to hold the body in balance for standing and walking.

Feet. Stand with the feet hip-width apart and very slightly turned out, with the weight evenly distributed between the balls of the feet and the heels.

Knees. The knees are at ease so they neither pull back tightly nor bend forwards.

Pelvis. You control the tilt of the pelvis so that it is not dropped too far down in front or lifted too far up (see p. 70).

Ribs. The ribcage is slightly lifted so that there is a good space between it and the hips. The upper back controls this movement.

Shoulders. The shoulders are down, away from the ears. Viewed from the side, they should be directly above the ankles.

Arms. Hang freely at your sides.

Neck. The back of the neck is lengthened upwards so that the chin is at about a right angle to the front of the neck.

Head. Feel you are lifting the crown of the head upwards. Ears directly above the shoulders.

This is a light, alive, alert stance and way of moving. Try not to sag anywhere. Half the secret is knowing what to do, and the other half is having the strength in your muscles, through practising the exercises, to enable you to do it. Refer back to the start of chapter 4 for a fuller explanation of good posture.

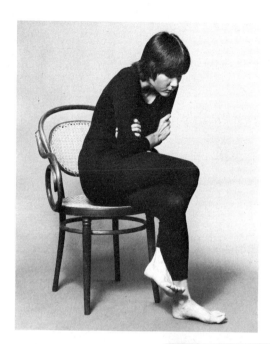

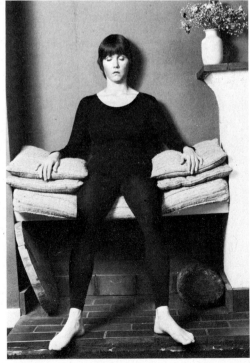

Physiological relaxation

It may seem odd in a book on movement to have a section devoted to something as apparently contradictory as relaxation. But in fact Laura Mitchell's method of physiological relaxation is based in itself on a series of orders for movement of the body, and as every athlete knows, relaxation is an essential part of activity. The method is fully explained in her book *Simple Relaxation*, but the following is a brief summary.

On the page opposite are a 'before' and an 'after' picture. The before picture shows the way stress and tension manifest themselves in the human body: body and head forward, shoulders raised, hands clenched, legs twisted round each other, foot held upwards. You will probably recognize some or all of these positions as habits of yours.

If you want to free your body from this wasteful and tiring pattern of stress, the technique of Physiological Relaxation as set out below will help you. But first there are some important facts to remember:

1. The brain must give a definite order that it recognizes will produce work.

2. The order that I have chosen for you to give to each joint will produce relaxation in the tense groups of muscles if you perform the movement exactly indicated by the words. When I say 'Pull your shoulders towards your feet' I mean *pull* not *drop*. Only voluntary activity will produce the reciprocal relaxation in the group opposite to the working group.

3. When I say 'Stop' I mean just that. You stop moving the part and you don't move it again. Don't try to substitute 'relax' for 'stop'. It won't help. You understand 'stop moving': do just that.

4. You register the feeling of the new position as accurately as you possibly can. This requires concentration, if you are not accustomed to it, but is otherwise extremely easy. I will try and assist you in this by describing the shape of your joint, the feelings you should get from your skin, e.g. in your finger-tips etc.

5. Remember you will be training yourself in *joint* and *skin* consciousness, not muscle consciousness, because that is the way the body works. There are no nerves recognizing muscle tension reach-

ing your upper brain, therefore you will not waste time and effort trying to feel it. You will be concentrating on the millions of sensory messages your conscious brain is constantly receiving from your joints and skin as your chosen muscles change their positions.

The orders are worded so that you can apply them to yourself whether lying on your back on the floor, sitting in a high-backed arm-chair, or sitting at a table with some cushions on it, onto which you lower arms and head. And of course a number of them can be done at any moment during the day, whether you are at a meeting, driving the car or whatever.

The sequence of orders is

1. arms
2. legs
3. body
4. head
5. breathing
6. face
7. mind

The orders in each joint are

1. move and feel
2. stop
3. feel

Check list of orders

ARMS

Shoulders
Order: Pull your shoulders towards your feet. STOP
Result: Feel your shoulders are further away from your ears. Your neck may feel longer.

Elbows
Order: Elbows out and open. STOP
Result: Feel your upper arms away from your body and the wide angle at your elbows. The weight of both arms should be resting on floor, chair arms, or pillows.

Hands
Order: Fingers and thumbs long and supported. STOP
Result: Feel your fingers and thumbs stretched out, separated, and touching support, nails on top. Especially feel your heavy thumbs.

LEGS

Hips
Order: Turn your hips outwards. STOP
Result: Feel your thighs rolled outwards. Knee-caps face outwards.

Knees
Order: Move slightly until comfortable if you wish. STOP
Result: Feel the resulting comfort in your knees.

Feet
Order: Push your feet away from your face, bending at the ankle. STOP
Result: Feel your dangling heavy feet.

BODY

Order: Push your body into the support. STOP
Result: Feel the contact of your body on the support.

HEAD

Order: Push your head into the support. STOP
Result: Feel the contact of your head on the support or pressure on the pillow.

BREATHING

Choose rate but try to keep it slow. Choose placing in routine before or after body and head, or when you feel your breathing rate slowing down. *Breathe in gently.* Expand the area in front above the waist, and between the angles of the ribcage, and raise your lower ribs upwards and outwards like the wings of a bird. Then *breathe out gently.* Feel your ribs fall downwards and inwards. Repeat once or at most twice.

FACE

Jaw

Order: Drag your jaw downwards. STOP

Result: Feel your separated teeth, heavy jaw, and loose lips – especially your lips.

Tongue

Order: Press your tongue downwards in your mouth. STOP

Result: Feel your loose tongue and slack gullet.

Eyes

Order: Close your eyes. STOP

Result: Feel your upper lids resting gently over your eyes, without any screwing up around the eyes. Enjoy the darkness.

Forehead

Order: Begin above eyebrows and think of smoothing gently up into your hair, over the top of your head and down the back of your neck. STOP

Result: Feel your hair move in the same direction.

MIND

Order: Either repeat the above sequence around the body, possibly more quickly. *Or* choose some subject which you will enjoy thinking about, and which has a sequence (song, prayer, poem, multiplication table, etc.). *Or* relive some past personal happy occasion. Let the mind play over these thoughts effortlessly, just to keep it occupied.

RETURN TO FULL ACTIVITY

Always stretch limbs and body in all directions and yawn. Do not hurry. Sit up slowly and wait for a minute or two before standing up.

7. Exercise in daily life

'Beauty from order springs.'
William King, 1663–1712
Art of Cooking

Some people do not wish to follow a set regime of exercises and yet would like to have the benefits of improved health and appearance which this would give them. This chapter is for them. It is also designed to provide back-up material for those who do perform the exercises in Chapters 5 and 6 but who want a change from the formal regime or are keen to continue their exercise throughout their day. It is perfectly possible to do the necessary movements on your own, in the course of your daily life, if you are willing to spend a bit of time understanding some of the essentials of bodily activity first, and then to carry out such activity with order and attention. All movements are useful but some are more useful than others.

In the bath

Have you ever thought of doing exercises in the bath? I do them every day. It is a pleasant relaxing place for busy people to linger in a little longer, and yet soothe their conscience by persuading themselves that they are still making good use of the time. It stops them doing the quick-time bath routine – in, scrub, out, dry – on to the next thing. I once used to have a telephone in the bathroom as well as the kitchen, bedroom, and sitting-room. That's how short of time I thought I was. But now I have learned, as I grow older, that really all that is quite silly, and that a gentle rest in a warm bath, with a few luxurious exercises to do, is sensible.

To be able to do these movements comfortably you may need to adjust your length to the length of your bath. I was fortunate, when I first put these movements together, that, with legs straight, my feet lay comfortably flat against the tap end of the bath, when my head was lying back against the top of the other end, while my neck rested on the rim. If the bath is very long it is rather a nuisance, and you have to do all the movements with your hips and knees bent and your feet on the floor of the bath to give you purchase. On the other hand the long bath has advantages for the disabled in that they can slither about on the smooth surface and just get some freedom of movement which is a special joy for them. If the bath is rather short for your full length, this is no great disadvantage. You just sit higher up. The water is a wonderful support, and although you are not completely weightless, much of the weight of your body and limbs is transferred to the bath and water. So every movement is easier to do. The smoothness of the surface is also a great help in moving. Then the sides of the bath and the tap end where your feet are, make an absolutely firm support on which to perform. You will find your head can get itself comfortable and supported on the other end. Some people favour a pillow but I find it gets damp and isn't easy to dry out. If you really need some neck support, use a rolled-up towel.

Of course I am not advocating anyone lying in a bath who has some condition which would make it dangerous. All these suggestions are for those with general good health, although it is also true that most chest troubles are helped by steamy warm conditions and rest. These exercises are of especial use to post-natal mums who should also add their pelvic floor muscle-lifting movements. If they have had stitches they will find the water soothing and they may care to add a handful of salt. Lingering in the bath gives them a much-needed rest and helps full recovery.

Old people can safely do these exercises and anyone with arthritis, especially of the spine, hips, knees, and feet, can get great benefit. Of course you do everything at your own pace and repeat just the number of times you find it pleasant. It is a good idea for those in pain, or who tire easily, to go through the regime as much as pleases them, then to have a rest in the water; listen to the radio perhaps, maybe eat an orange, and then again do a few movements. I always have a basket of oranges and grapefruit beside the bath and a fruit knife. You just dip your sticky fingers into your outsize finger bowl: another ingredient in the general feeling of well-being which it is so important to try to develop, if you are often in pain or have difficulty trying to get about. An oasis of pleasure in a long, difficult, frustrating day of pain, is worth more than all the pep talks

of the well-meaning. So encourage yourself with all the small ameni-
ties that a bathroom can offer; plants, coloured towels, a soft cover
for the lavatory seat, and, if possible, have a coloured ceiling – either
paper or paint. Remember that, if you are going to be there for ten
to fifteen minutes, your eyes will be directed to the ceiling.

It is often a good idea to vary the timing of a movement, slow
and then quick, because muscles will always respond to the demands
put on them for movement and timing; this keeps them strong and
active, and ready to respond to your needs from day to day. Usually
it is best to begin with slow thorough movements until you get the
feeling properly of what is happening in your joints and then repeat
the same performance rather more quickly, even carelessly. You may
also feel a pull on the fibrous tissue (the scaffolding of muscle) on
the side opposite to the working part. This sensation depends upon
how much these muscles have shortened, and should never be forced.
Gentle movement is the best way to coax things back to normal.
Never at any time give yourself pain; pain is a warning sign and,
to my mind, means you are doing something uncongenial to your
body and you should stop at once. You may care to try the same
movement again very carefully; then, if the pain has not recurred,
you can continue. Never perform any relaxation technique in the
bath because of the very real danger of going to sleep, and then slipping under the water.

So here are the movements. Just do them in any order you like
with rests in between. Select those suitable for you and ignore the
others. I have included movements for the whole body.

TUMMY

Remembering the formation of the muscles of the abdominal wall
pp. 56–58) we must do a forward shortening of them, a side shortening, a twisting shortening, and a sustained flattening.

Forward shortening. Lean back so that your head and neck are resting
on the end of the bath. Plant your feet firmly on the floor of the
bath so that your hips and knees are bent. If, for any reason, you
cannot comfortably do this, just keep your legs stretched out. Bend
your arms so that your elbows are touching the sides of the bath
and each hand rests on the knob of the projecting pelvic bone at

each side of the curve of your tummy. You have now a firm base
for your feet and a firm support for your chest, head, and neck. Roll
your pelvis gently and firmly so that the bony part in front comes
towards your nose; at the same time you will find your spinal bones
at the back, at the level of your waist, are now nearly touching or
are touching the floor of the bath. You have rocked your pelvis up
at the front and so of course it goes down at the back, and the front
of your tummy has flattened. Now just let go and you will feel your
pelvis roll back again; if you like, slightly arch your back so the front
of your pelvis falls even further down. Then return to the first movement. Don't hold your breath. To stop this, sing to yourself as you
move, or breathe out when you roll your pelvis up in front and
breathe in when you roll it downwards. That means you breathe out
always when you flatten your tummy. Never allow your breathing
to push your tummy forwards forcibly. This only stretches it and
no-one wants a stretched abdominal wall, although many people
stretch theirs by doing abdominal exercises wrongly. Repeat as often
as you feel comfortable. This movement shortens and strengthens
all the front of your tummy muscles. It also lubricates the joints of
your low back, and your hip joints.

Side shortening. Keep your head and neck supported, your hands
on the projecting pelvic bones on either side, and your legs either
bent up or long, as you wish. Now pull one side of your pelvis up
towards your armpit, and your waist will tuck in at that side. Push
it down again and pull it up on the other side. You will feel your
bottom swivel sideways on the smooth bath surface and your hands
resting on your pelvis will also feel that swinging from side to side.
Continue to do this smooth sideways movement as long as it gives
you pleasure. You will probably feel movement in your spine on
the right and left side of your waist because this is where the movement is taking place, so that as well as strengthening the sides of
your abdominal muscles, you also strengthen your back muscles
at either side alternately. You can't choose exactly which muscles
will work, because your brain can't do this. You can only choose
which movement you perform, and all the muscles which can con-
veniently further this movement will come into action. This is why
the starting position and what you tell yourself to do is so important.
In this way only can you control which muscles will work.

Twisting shortening. Keep your head and neck still supported, your elbows against the sides of the bath and your hands across your chest. Straighten one leg and press the toes firmly against the wall of the bath below the taps, then curl the tops of the toes of the other foot around that ankle or heel. Now you twist your pelvis around towards the side of the straight leg. This is easy because of the fixed points of your toes at one end and your head and chest at the other. You don't need to create a great wave of water that will swamp the bathroom floor; a steady firm twisting movement is what is wanted. Once again your bottom moves easily on the smooth floor of the bath and much of your weight is being supported both by the bath and the water in it. Thus you will probably find you can do the twisting with great satisfaction several times. You then change the position of your feet so that you can twist in the opposite direction and you get a magnificent feeling of freedom and movement. This action is taking place in your hip joints and the joints of your upper spine close to your ribs. Therefore the muscles working are those which cross your tummy and your back in an oblique direction. You are tightening up all the muscles which support your innards and your spine, and hold you in a well-balanced, good-looking upright position when you stand up.

Flattening shortening. Your head and neck should be supported by the back of the bath, your hands lying loosely on lower ribs at either side so that the finger-tips just touch in front in the little hollow between the angle of the ribs. Breathe in easily and lift the ribs sideways. You will feel them rise upwards under your hands (see p. 73), and feel the little hollow under your finger-tips fill forward slightly because you are using your diaphragm. Although it only descends about one inch, this is enough to increase the pressure within the abdomen. Do not arch your back at all or push your belly forwards. It should be a gentle, easy movement forward in front above your waist and an uplifting sideways of the ribs. Now blow out easily and as you do so, pull your tummy back as strongly and firmly as you can, and think of narrowing your waist. Do not try to force all your breath out because of course you can't. Your lungs are never empty of air until you have breathed out your last breath on this earth. Just concentrate on the feeling of shortening, narrowing pressure all around your tummy and let the air stream comfortably outwards.

Then hold a moment and repeat the whole process. There must be no gasping or prolonged breath-holding; it should all feel natural and pleasant. Repeat only twice, have a rest, and then do other movements.

BACK

Lie with legs stretched out if possible, feet against the tap end of the bath, and head against the other end. Elbows rest against sides of bath. Begin low in the back and hollow your back right up the whole length of it till you are only supported on your bottom and the back of your head. Stay like this for a few seconds breathing easily, and turn your legs outwards, pressing back your thighs on the floor of the bath. Next slacken your legs and slowly lay your spine back again bit by bit, beginning from the low back and progressing to the head. After that you may enjoy lifting your head and pulling it forwards. If so, roll up so that you are directing your nose in towards your chest. In this way you give a little stretch to your back muscles which will enable you more easily to repeat the arching, if you want, later. If you do repeat, when you have done the full arch backwards, try to draw your shoulder blades strongly together as you press your head finally backwards. This time keep your nose facing forwards and hook the back of your skull onto the bath end. Repeat as often as feels comfortable, and be sure to breathe easily or sing throughout.

NECK

You have of course used the muscles at the back of your neck when you extended your head backwards, thus hollowing your neck. You have also used the muscles at the front of your neck when you tipped your head forwards towards your breast-bone. But there is more you can do to preserve the length of your neck and to lubricate its seven joints more precisely.

Starting position. Sit up either with your legs straight out or bent, as you prefer. Place your forearms along the edges of the bath and grasp the sides with your hands so that the weight of each arm is on the bath (see p. 27). Pull your shoulder blades together two, three or four times, then draw your elbows as far back along the bath tops as may be comfortable, loosening your hand grips to do so.

Stop doing this, leave the arms where they have arrived, and again hold on with your hands. You have now a good foundation from which to work the neck muscles, some of which are attached to your collar bones and shoulder blades. Both these bones are now in a corrected pulled-back position. Their weight is always tending to drag them forwards and slump onto the chest, due to the pull of gravity.

Three-point pull. Keep you nose facing straight forwards, and attempt to stretch the top of your head to the ceiling, at the same time pulling the tops of your shoulders down towards the water. I call this a 'three-point pull' (see picture on p. 70). Stop. Feel your head balanced in this corrected position and that your neck has lengthened. This is in fact true. The natural curve of your seven neck bones is forwards, and with the great weight of your five or six kilogram (twelve pounds) head sitting on the top, pressing downwards, the curve tends to get accentuated and shorter. The correction reduces this and allows the seven vertebrae (spinal bones) and intervertebral discs to move more freely, instead of being pressed closely together.

Now you can safely and pleasantly bend your head forwards and downwards, then take it upwards, and when the top of your head is uppermost again, do another little stretch, and then tilt it as far back as you like. This should be performed as slowly and fully as possible. Finally bring your head up, so that it balances evenly, facing forwards with your ear above the point of your shoulder. *Never* move your head on your neck as an exercise, without doing the stretching, or else you just grind the bones on each other – the worst movement is to roll your heavy head around your neck without any stretching movement whatever, as I see so many people doing. It is asking for bone or cartilage damage and tends to make your head settle still further into your neck when you have finished the torture.

Starting position. Now lean back and place your head on the back wall of the bath. You are going to do the next neck movements without the weight of your head. Repeat the three-point pull as your head rests there, and put your arms back in the warm water.

Head turning. Now just roll your head to right and then left, slowly, each time trying to get a little further around so that you would be showing a perfect profile if you were looked at from the front. You may like to let your head rest for a few minutes at the side and then do the same at the other side; then you can finish with a fairly swift movement from side to side if you like. Since your head is supported this is quite safe. When you feel like it, stop, do the three-point pull and finish with that.

Head side bending. You have stretched your neck without the weight of your head, you have bent it forwards and extended it backwards, and you have turned it from side to side, so all your straight and oblique muscles have been working. The last movement is to bend your head to the side while it rests against the bath end, so that you bring your ear down towards your shoulder. You must not twist at all this time. Your nose faces forward continuously. Straighten up, do your three-point pull, and then bend to the other side, trying to get your other ear onto that shoulder. When you have had enough side bending, finish with a final three-point pull. Then you have earned another rest.

ARMS

You have already done a good deal in the way of pulling your collar bones and shoulder blades backwards and downwards away from your ears. You have also pulled your shoulder blades together when doing the back exercises, so you have considerably improved on the usual unfortunate slack position of these bones, when they fall forwards. All you have to do now is to strengthen the surrounding muscles and lubricate your shoulder joints. These are naturally very loose joints. Did you know your shoulder joint can be pulled out about 2 inches (5 cms) quite safely because it is so loose? The part of the shoulder blade that makes the socket is much smaller than the top of the arm bone which forms the other part of the shoulder joint. For this reason the shoulder joint will dislocate very easily if you fall on it when you are young. You should never lift a child by one of his upstretched arms because you could easily pull the arm out of its socket.

To tether the arm bone against the socket there is a very intricate arrangement of tendons winding around the bones. This usually works very satisfactorily but as we get older we tend not to use the arms so freely, the whole area may then get stiff and, as it were, glued together while the muscles weaken. Any injury to the hand or fore-arm may mean that we do not use the arm on that side fully and therefore may develop a stiff weakened shoulder as well as the other injury.

Outward rotation. Exercise one arm at a time. Most baths are placed against a wall but you will find the movements can be done by the arm on the wall side if you sit well over to give yourself room. Place the elbow on the side of the bath. Place your hand palm down onto the bath edge and then, keeping a right angle between forearm and elbow, lift your hand and forearm up and back as near to the vertical as possible. You can give it several little extra pushes backwards if you like. This strengthens the muscles used to rotate your shoulder joint outwards, which is what you are doing. These muscles help to raise your arm above your head. Repeat as often as you wish. This is quite a powerful exact movement which selects the muscles that turn your arm outwards at the shoulder joint (Lateral Rotators), so don't overdo it.

Inward rotation. Place the back of your hand on your waist behind you, then push it up between your shoulder blades. Continue this up-and-down pumping movement a few times, trying to get your finger-tips further up each time. This movement helps you put your arm behind you into a jacket sleeve. Afterwards, either put your arm back in the water for a little rest and warmth, or proceed to the final activity.

Arm lifting. Place the elbow on the side of the bath with the fore-arm bent up so that your hand rests on your shoulder. Now raise your elbow towards your ear and then lower it down onto the bath edge. Wag it up and down like this, gradually increasing the action. Finally, you put your forearm over the top of your head, and the side of your upper arm is touching your ear. Hold it there and straighten your elbow so your hand goes up towards the ceiling. Now repeat the same sideways up-and-down movement with a straight arm. You have by this means increased the difficulty of the exercise (see p. 27) so only do this if you find you can with ease. It will strengthen the muscles if you do, but you, alone, can decide if you feel ready for it. Take a rest. Now sit near to the other side of the bath and repeat all the above with the other arm.

Arm circling. Finally sit in the middle of the bath, put both hands on your shoulders, and make the points of your elbows turn around in as wide a circle as possible, first forwards and then backwards. You might like to stretch both hands up to the ceiling after that. See that your upper arms touch your ears as evidence of loose yet strong shoulder joints.

LEGS

If your hips, knees, ankles, or feet are weak or painful, perhaps after an injury, this is an ideal way to help the circulation in the warm water, loosen the joints, and strengthen the muscles that support them. Movement is useful – for increasing circulation, for increasing muscle power, and for preserving joint mobility.

Hip and knee bending. Lie with head and neck supported and feet on tap wall of bath, palms of hands under thighs. It is better to move one leg at a time. Curl your toes downwards and firmly bring your toes up the floor of the bath towards your bottom so that you bend your ankle, your knee, and your hip joint. Continue the movement as fully as possible. You may have to give a little help with the supporting hand under your thigh, but this must not force the leg up. Your hand is only there to relieve some of the weight which, of course, the water is already doing. You may find it comfortable to move both legs at once with the knees pressed together, as each leg supports the other. But if you have more movement in one leg than the other, move one at a time. When you have scratched your toes along the bath actively pushing your leg upwards, try to bend your knee and hip just a little more so your knee comes towards your nose and foot comes off the floor of the bath. Keep the leg in this final position for a few moments. By using this positive scratching movement of your toes along the bottom of the bath and then bending your knee and hip, you force the muscles on the back of your lower leg and thigh to work hard and finally the muscles that bend the hip work with them. Muscles work best in collaboration with groups with which they normally associate during activity (see p. 42). Now just let your leg go easily back into the water.

Hip and knee strengthening – one. When you have had enough of the scratching and bending-up movement, you now do the straightening out, first one leg then the other, or both together. Bend your ankle so that your toes come towards your face as strongly as you can. Keep it in this position and drive your heel down onto the floor, and then strongly towards the end of the bath, so that you straighten out your knee as fully as possible, still keeping the foot turned upwards. Your heels will finally come off the floor of the bath. You have now strengthened the muscles on the front of your lower leg and the front of your thigh. Finally turn your knees outwards (this is really rotation of the hips) while you press your thighs onto the floor of the bath; you will have strengthened your buttock muscles also. You need all these muscles strong to stand up straight. As you lie having a rest with legs out straight, just roll your legs outwards and inwards so that your feet turn as far as possible out and in each time (medial and lateral rotators of hip joints).

Hip and knee strengthening – two. Keep your toes facing the ceiling and your knees fully extended, open your legs so that the sides of your feet press strongly against the sides of the bath. Do this several times singing or counting as you do so, so that you don't hold your breath. The muscles on the outside of each hip (abductors of hip joints) really do need to be kept strong, because they support you and steady your pelvis when you are walking.

Ankles. Either sit up or lie back as you wish. Raise one knee and hold both your hands under the thigh so that your hands steady the weight of your leg and your foot is suspended in the water. Now turn your foot around very slowly, making a big circle with your great toe. Be sure you get the maximum movement in all four directions – up, in, down and out. Then reverse and make a circle in the opposite direction. Repeat the whole process with your other leg.

Feet. These are usually best worked together. Lie in usual position with both feet against the wall at the tap end of the bath. The water should be deep enough to cover the whole of the feet and toes. Bend and stretch your toes several times. Now try to spread the toes so you make spaces between them, then close them up. Continue opening and closing. Some people cannot do this at all, especially if they wear tight stockings or shoes, but keep trying; the warm water helps.

Finally, keep your toes stretched out forwards and hump up the middle of your feet so that you have now drawn the pads of your toes towards your heels, with the toes remaining straight. You will find you have arched your feet in two directions, longways and across the top, where your toes begin. You have strengthened all the small muscles of the feet, preserved your arches, and hastened the circulation around all the tiny joints in the feet. Stop and then repeat several times. This should make much happier feet for you to stand and walk on.

FINAL MOVEMENT

You perform this gradually and fully in your own time, adding each movement in sequence and holding it as you add the next. Press your feet against the corners of the tap end of the bath, then press your thighs against the floor of the bath, then extend your whole spine, then press your head against the other end of the bath with your nose facing forwards, then push your elbows against the sides of the bath, and pull your shoulder blades together. You are now practising all the movements, and therefore strengthening all the muscles, that you use to stand upright. You will probably find this a very satisfying thing to do. So repeat it once or twice if you want to – be sure you don't hold your breath or hold the final position too long, because it really is hard work. Just enjoy the feeling of straightening yourself out. Have a rest.

GETTING IN AND OUT OF THE BATH

If you have any difficulty getting in or out of the bath, this is what to do. Sit on a small towel on the edge of the bath, with your back to it. Hold onto the side of the bath, then swivel sideways towards the tap end – this is very easy to do on the towel – till one knee is touching the side of the bath. Have your knees touching each other. Now carefully lift the leg nearest to the bath into it – with assistance if necessary. Then lift in the other leg. You are now sitting on the side with your feet in the water. Now lean across and put your hand on the far side of the bath so that you face the taps. Grasp the near side with your other hand and lower yourself into the water. If you need assistance be sure you direct it yourself. If you find standing up difficult, the safest thing to do is to turn around and get onto your hands and knees, then you can easily hold onto the side and so stand up. Whatever you do, take it slowly and carefully. You must feel safe on every move before you attempt the next one. If you have the slightest fear that you will not be able to get out of the bath, do not get into it in the first place, unless there is someone else in the house and you have left the bathroom door unlocked.

In the shower

You may have a shower instead of a bath, but you can still do your extra activity there. You may be showering because this is your preference, or because you are too unsure of yourself to get into a bath. In either case you have a chance to do movements that are most valuable for your health and posture, and which everyone is apt to miss in daily living. Warm up between exercises with a warm shower or try doing some of the movements with the water running over you. Experiment to find what you like best, and select the movements as you wish.

Let us hope you make a habit of scrubbing yourself all over as vigorously as possible with a loofah – stimulation of the skin being so important in maintaining 'feedback' to the brain that is part of all activity (p. 38). You also rub off the dead skin always accumulating on the surface. As you sway, twist, and turn, do so as thoroughly and yet as quickly as you can. Quick, deft movements keep your brain in living co-operation with your body, whereas skimpy, slovenly movements cause a slowing down of receptive sensitivity. Even if you have to sit on a chair or stool under the shower, you can still do all that. One wants to beware of slowing down every movement just because one part has become slow or awkward. For example, try to keep washing your own back and feet, even if you are disabled and it is difficult. Anyone helping you will always want to do these. 'It's quicker' they say. So you reply like the Chinaman 'and what shall I do with the time saved?' Probably nothing – and meantime you have handed over part of the responsibility for your own body to someone else: a very bad bargain.

If you are safe standing on one leg, be sure you do so, when you attend to the other leg and foot. This strengthens the muscles of your standing leg and foot, and the muscles of your tummy and back as you sway. It also keeps the balance centres in your brain receptive, in dealing with changes in posture. If you lean against a support you miss all these useful nerve sensations informing the brain of alteration in shape and pressure. The answering responses in motor nerves telling muscles what to do automatically, are therefore not practised as they might be.

ARMS

Do the bath exercises for arms (pp. 178–180) as quickly and thoroughly as possible. When you finish with the upwards stretch, straighten your knees, rise up on your toes, and elongate the complete length of your spine, at the same time driving the top of your head towards the ceiling, with chin drawn in. This gives a lovely feeling of competence and control of your upright posture.

TUMMY AND BACK

Spread your feet slightly and grip the rubber mat, or roughened tiles, with your toes. Now slightly bend your hips and knees and, holding this leg position firmly, tilt your pelvis forward and backwards, then from side to side, and finally twist it from right to left and vice versa. Do all these movements fairly vigorously. All the time your top half should remain facing forwards and to fix this you can hold onto the wall or curtain supports if you need to, and if they are strong enough. Then you can finish by doing the circular pelvic movement which you may have seen being performed by eastern dancers. This should be rather slower so as to achieve as full a circle as possible. These pleasurable exercises will keep your tummy flat and neat, I hope – remember that double layer of fat under the skin (p. 55). Be sure you sing, shout, or count as you do all this, so that you don't hold your breath.

ANKLES AND FEET

Stand on one leg, and, holding your other leg with both hands around your thigh, perform the ankle circling. Then with both feet on the mat, do the toe exercises, and then hump up the foot arches as described in the bath exercises on pp. 181–182.

LEGS

The good old-fashioned 'heel raising, knee bending' exercise is a most useful one because it strengthens and tightens the muscles of your bottom, fronts of thighs, and the muscles at the outside and back of your lower legs. Do not bend lower than you are sure you can recover from. You will gradually, in time, be able to sink lower down, as the muscles strengthen.

Put your hands on your hips and stand sideways, so that you can lift one leg up to the side and slightly backwards at the hip joint. Raise it slowly, with the foot facing forward and the knee bent a little; immediately you feel your pelvis begin to tilt sideways under your hand; hold your leg where it is, and then lower it slowly to the ground. This will limit training to hip movement and hip muscle control and cut out spinal ones. You strengthen the muscles on the outside and back of your thigh and make it neat and strong. You have now exercised all your leg muscles. You need them to be strong so as to be able to balance on one leg – something you do with every step you take.

Remember what you are trying to do is just lubricate your joints, strengthen your muscles, keep your brain active in response to demand for movement, and enjoy yourself. There is no point in wearing yourself out, or trying to show off, unless you are trying to save water and shower with a friend.

In bed

All the bath exercises can be performed in bed, with a few differences. These comparatively weightless exercises are of use to all manner of people, young and old, but of course you must never exercise if you are confined to bed with any infection. They are only for those in normal health or perhaps convalescing. When you are out of bed for a certain time each day, you may prefer to augment the time you spend up with these bed exercises.

Muscles work best in short bursts of real activity. It isn't much use doing bed exercises in a casual manner for a longer time. So decide yourself what suits you best. You may vary from day to day depending on how you feel and why you are working in bed – one to two minutes' activity in every hour is a very safe plan. You could work for five minutes sometimes but you will find this is a long time if you are working hard. Don't attempt to exercise every area each time. You are supposed to be enjoying the activity, so choose which bits of your body need extra attention. Then, in your next bout you either repeat these exercises, or deal with another part of your body as may be necessary.

POSITIONS IN BED

Sitting. You may have gathered by now, because I nag about it so much, that when you are resting in bed you must have your head, and especially your neck, supported by pillows. The important fact to remember is that your head weighs about 12 pounds (5 kilos) and therefore sitting up in bed while still holding it up is very tiring. So tuck a little sausage-shaped pillow into your neck and see you have some other pillow just behind your head to receive its weight. I use a larger square pillow which supports both back and head. Press back into this, then stop pressing, and leave your head lying on it.

If you want luxurious comfort, have a pillow under each upper arm, or you can get a pillow shaped like a large horseshoe, which is a most comfortable support for head, neck, back, and arms, all at once. Of course all bed clothes should be loose at all times, never tucked in tightly. This encourages movement, even during sleep. People sometimes ask what position they should choose, in which to sleep. The answer is whatever is comfortable, and which helps you to go off to sleep. It is normal to move during sleep.

Lying. This is the other position for bed exercises. If possible lie with no pillows at all. You may find you are more comfortable with the small sausage pillow under your neck and if your low back complains, do not put a pillow into its hollow; instead, put the pillow under your thighs and I think you will find this relieves the discomfort in your back.

EXERCISES SITTING (in addition to bath exercises)

Legs. Legs tend to lie close together and to cross over, so whenever you think about it, part your legs and just leave them apart. You will be surprised to find they always come in together again, by themselves, so there is no need to do this movement.

When you have the legs apart and straight out, roll the whole leg so that you turn the knee-cap as fully as possible inwards and outwards. The outside of your foot should rest on the sheet as you turn it outwards, but when you turn it in you will only get your foot about halfway down to the sheet. You have ten muscles which turn your hip out and only three very small ones that turn it in. The hip-joint formation also favours outward rotation.

The next exercise you can perform with one leg or both at once, as you wish. Bend your knees; place your feet flat on the sheet and bend all your toes into it; then continue this scratching movement against the sheet and the resistance of the mattress, so that you propel the legs up the bed with your heels moving towards your bottom. Keep close contact against the sheet so that your muscles have to work really hard to move your feet along. When you have your knees at a right angle, press hard down into the mattress and you will feel your spine extend. This is a reflex action, called the plantar reflex (see p. 38), and by keeping this working you are helping yourself to keep upright when you are out of bed.

Now tip your toes up into the air, at the same time bending the feet up at the ankles and driving your heels hard into the mattress. In this position and in this manner, thrust them right down the bed, till your knees are quite straight, and your toes pointing to the ceiling. Press the backs of your thighs into the bed and let your legs separate and turn outwards. Again, if you wish you can extend your spine at the same time, so that your head presses back strongly into the pillows and your elbows press into the mattress on either side. Keep singing or counting; never hold your breath. Now rest for a little; you deserve it because you have worked all the muscles of your legs hard, and the muscles of your back. So when you stand up you should feel splendid.

Arms. You perform the arm movements either sitting up or lying flat. It depends upon the position and width of your bed, whether you can use both arms together, or separately. Use the bath exercises. If you find some small alterations necessary, I leave you to arrange these yourself.

Tummy. These movements are all the same as in the bath except for the twisting. The pelvic tilting and side bending you will find rather more difficult because you are not lying on such a slippery surface, but the resistance makes your muscles work harder.

Here is how to do twisting in bed and still keep warm. Lie flat, face up. Spreadeagle your feet to the two corners of the lower end of the bed. If yours is a very narrow one, put the feet over the edge at each side. Now just slightly raise your head and bring the right hand up to it. Twist to the left side, looking round and placing the palm of your right hand onto the mattress, as close to your body as possible. Don't hold your breath. It is often a good idea to blow out as you twist, and then to breathe in as you come back to your starting position again. Repeat as often as you wish, and then twist in the opposite direction.

Back. Try what you can comfortably do of the bath exercises. There is one extra: *Five holes in the bed*. This works like magic for strengthening backs. I have been recommending it to patients for many years, and have used it myself with great comfort and success. Lie flat on the bed. You are going to push your heels, head, and elbows or hands (as you prefer) into the mattress. You are *not* to anchor these parts *on* the mattress and heave your back off it. You are to work to make holes *into* the mattress, beginning with any of the five parts you prefer. Once you have got them pushing hard, you maintain this push and add the next. Your spine will gradually extend slightly. It should be extremely hard work, as you are working against the resistance of the springs of the mattress, and it will strengthen your back muscles powerfully and completely safely. Sing or count as you do this or you will hold your breath. Repeat once only.

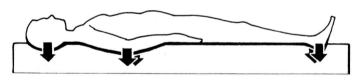

'Five holes in the bed'

In the kitchen

The kitchen can be a very suitable place in which to practise exercise. In the pages for the over sixties (pp. 197–198) you will find suggestions to make work in the kitchen either easier or more difficult, as you may prefer. We all have to wait for a kettle to boil, for something to cook that needs stirring from time to time,. or for the oven to heat up. We can use the time for a quick bout of activity.

Try especially doing arm stretching above the head (p. 180), spinal extension (p. 176), and the three-point pull for the head and neck (p. 70). These will all help to counteract the bending forward which all cooking entails. We are so apt to go from one job to another without correcting ourselves out of this dangerous position. It is dangerous because gravity is always pulling us down in any case, and when we sit and peel vegetables, prepare any dish, or perhaps clean something, we enhance this by looking downwards all the time, while our hands work in front of us. So if we quickly, or slowly and luxuriously, stretch in the opposite direction up and out, we stop ourselves getting overtired by holding the forward positions. We may also stop our joints becoming deformed.

You will find you can do the four necessary movements to reduce your tummy – pelvic tilting, pelvic twisting, side bending, and strong retractions (pp. 56–58) very thoroughly in two minutes, if you go about it briskly. It's a good sequence habit to develop – put on the kettle, reduce your tummy size, make the tea.

Much has been written about making work habits and gadgets like an ironing board suit the person using them. This is called ergonomics and the science should be applied in your kitchen just as it is in a modern factory. For example if you are not very tall, you may find it more convenient to stand on a strong box at the sink, rather than overstretch to use it. If, however, you are tall, you may find it suits you better to put the box inside the sink, and perch a basin on the top. Then you won't have to stoop down uncomfortably to reach it. Give it a bit of thought.

Many kitchens have all the working surfaces at exactly the same height. Do they suit you? Do they suit every other member of the family who uses the kitchen? Could you arrange to have some higher and some lower, to suit everyone and to give your body, especially your spine, a variety of positions in which to work? Remember your body reacts well to change. It doesn't like being fixed and forced to work continuously without relief in any one position.

Often the oven is so positioned that there is no surface at hand on which to place the dish that you are putting into or removing from it. This means you may have to carry a heavy, very hot casserole or roasting pan across to a table, which can be tiring and dangerous. Try to see that you have a heatproof surface beside the oven and that your oven door opens downwards, so that it can be used as a tray on which to rest the dish for inspection or basting. Exercise in the kitchen should be by design not accident.

Scrubbing a kitchen floor on hands and knees is now frowned upon as old-fashioned. It is, in fact, a very useful back and tummy exercise. This position enhances the natural curves of the vertebral column – forward in the neck, backwards in the upper back (dorsal), and forwards in the low back (lumbar). Look at the side view of the skeleton on page 50. The only disadvantage is the pressure on the knee joints, so always kneel on a bit of sponge rubber. If you put it in a polythene bag it won't get damp. Then happily wiggle your back and your bottom as much as you can while you work. Take large sweeps with your arm and try to work with alternate arms. Then wringing out a cloth is wonderful activity to make rounded strong forearms. Of course use a lightweight bucket and always bend your hips and knees and keep your back straight as you lift it. This reduces the size of your bottom and thighs. Sitting back onto your heels and straightening up again a few times will also work your quadriceps muscles in front of your thighs and help to make them a good shape. If you sing as you work you'll also increase your breathing capacity. As you are making yourself more healthy and beautiful you certainly have something to sing about.

Whether you are man or woman, give some thought to all the jobs you do around the house, and see if you are using your body sensibly to do them, or if you are abusing it. Remember it is your most precious tool and treat it with as much consideration as your sewing machine or carpentry outfit. It will repay correct use by debeloping greater efficiency via stronger, more agile muscles, more mobile joints, and better use of blood and oxygen. Give your body the respect it is due, and it will serve you well.

In the office

Your desk should be the correct height for you to work at comfortably, neither too low so that your back is curved forwards, nor too high so that it strains your arms. Your chair should be stable: some typists' chairs which sway about are lethal to human backs. If the chair back is tall enough for you to rest your head against it sometimes, you will be doing the seven joints in your neck a great service, by giving them a break from carrying the weight of your head. Then you can do the three-point pull and roll your head from side to side, and bend it sideways occasionally. This undoes the pressure on these joints safely and comfortably.

If you sit a great deal, try standing sometimes, instead, to take a phone call. Brace your knees strongly, stretch your spine, hold your head high, and you'll give yourself some posture training while working. It also makes you feel more alert than sitting in a bundle all day. Try, too, to look up to the ceiling above your head for a minute after you have been gazing downwards for some time.

If you like isometric exercises, you can do these at your desk but be sure you don't hold your breath and only do a limited session. Intersperse with some free movements.

If you have to talk to colleagues in the same building, why not go and see them sometimes – by stairs not lift – rather than use the phone? Can you run up the stairs?

Vary your activities whenever possible and try not to sit longer than half an hour at any time. Try to regard your desk as a temporary work bench, rather than an anchor to which you are bound. Go and do some filing, or walk about as you dictate, for a change. If you get stuck in one of those long meetings, at least move your legs about and wriggle your toes inside your shoes. This is a great help in quickening your circulation back to your heart and so to your brain. You can also take a couple of diaphragmatic breaths – no more than two – as further assistance to the blood stream. I hope you also practise relaxation at your desk when you feel yourself getting into the stress position (see p. 167).

In the garden

The professional gardener learns to pace himself to work and weather. The amateur would learn a lot by studying his way of working. It all looks deceptively simple, but then so does a pirouette by a well-trained ballerina on the points of her toes. The answer is planning, timing, and above all practical experience.

LIFTING, LAYING, PUSHING, AND CARRYING

Use your legs. The muscles in them are large, strong, and rather coarse in fibre, especially the buttock muscles, and stand up well to heavy work. The hip joints are very safely constructed to move in all directions and are supported all round by strong ligaments. This is so different from the rather more delicate muscles controlling the finer joints of the spinal column. So always put the brunt of any heavy weight you may be moving or carrying through your legs by keeping your back still, and making your hips take the strain. Then if you want to turn, move your feet first. Lift and lay by bending hips and knees with a straight back; keep the object close to you, and when possible, put it on your head or back to carry, rather than clasping it in your arms and humping it about with your back rounded.

If you only garden very infrequently, limit yourself to half an hour at a time at any one task. When you have to bend forward planting out or weeding remember to keep breathing easily. If you find you have held your breath at a crucial moment, just breathe out gently. Get into the habit of easy diaphragmatic breathing (pp. 73–75). Alternate the forward bent position with stretching out in all directions. Straighten yourself up completely and then take a rest. Have you noticed the professional gardener leaning on his spade? He wasn't wasting his time. He was saving his spinal column from injury. It is we amateurs who work away in a frenzy, and rush round the garden like a hurricane, who damage ourselves.

TOOLS AND PLANNING

Choose tools with great care. Money spent on stainless steel ones means you have an easily cleaned, sharp surface instead of a soil-encrusted heavy object to heave about. There are many modern tools that save back-breaking labour so, having assessed your requirements, search out what will help you enjoy your gardening, and return to it with pleasure. You want to spend your energy on the actual gardening work, not wrestling with inadequate tools.

On each gardening expedition, collect what you think you may need in a lightweight basket. Use foam rubber in a nylon bag for kneeling on; use lightweight plastic bags for transporting rubbish, peat, or compost. If you use a barrow, get as far forward between the shafts as you can, so that you are absolutely erect and your head is up. Then holding the handles easily with both hands and straight elbows, push the weight forward from your hips. If you haven't a barrow to shift weights, drag them behind you with straight arms holding your head and back upright. Your elbow joints are so made that when they are straightened out, the bones lock together. This saves muscle work and danger of damage.

Try to vary your jobs; plan before you go out what you will do, so that you have some kneeling, perhaps for weeding or transplanting, some bending and twisting, perhaps for tying up or pruning, some carrying or scattering, perhaps compost or fertilizer, so that you don't overdo any single kind of movement. And don't do more than you planned: it is very tempting.

Digging must be learned from experts and only done in short spells by the amateur. 'They *will* try to turn over the world in one afternoon' said one professional gardener. Beware of working in cold winds; muscles do not like a Siberian draught when they are working. Wear layers of lightweight warm clothing, suitable boots or shoes, and often a wool cap in winter. Above all stop when you are tired. Your movements then become awkward, and though you may not notice how clumsy you have become, you may easily hurt yourself. Do remember to leave time and energy to put all your tools away safely and dispose of the rubbish. Don't work on till the last bit of your energy is exhausted at this unaccustomed labour; this causes accidents.

Dentist and hairdresser

This section may be called 'dentist and hairdresser' but what I have to say applies to all those whose work involves either a lot of standing or a lot of leaning forward, or both. The common enemies that I have my sights on are varicose veins, neck and back trouble, and general tiredness. They do not discriminate; both lathe operators and stockbrokers fall prey.

Hairdressers stand all day, and are usually leaning forward as well. They are prone to varicose veins as is anyone who stands all day at work. The flow of blood upwards from the legs is the most difficult area of the circulation, as it has to climb against gravity back to the heart. The action of muscles and the movement of joints normally assist this, but if they are not being used very much, the blood is apt to pool in the little pockets (valves) inside the veins and thus stretch the walls (p. 79). To counteract this, hairdressers should form the habit of bending the toes and opening them out frequently inside their shoes as they stand. The muscles working in the feet and the backs of the lower legs squeeze the blood upwards. If they would also sometimes rise onto their toes once or twice quickly they may save months of misery from aching legs.

If veins are once stretched in width they never recover, and you may have to wear elastic stockings for the rest of your life, or have an operation. Walk part of the way to work if you can, and walk about whenever possible during the day. During lunch-time put your feet up level with your hips, or slightly higher, if you can. Sit down and rest sometimes, rather than stand around when you are not busy. Choose shoes that support your insteps, or your feet will spread by your weight continuously passing through them, without much muscular activity to support the small bones of your feet. It is a good idea to have a change of shoes during the day.

To counteract the continuous forward bending position be sure the clients' chairs are high enough for you to attend to them with the minimum of leaning down. It is a great help if trolleys for rollers, brushes, etc. are higher rather than lower. Remember you will be repeating identical hand and arm movements hundreds of times a day, so do rest the working muscles often by activating their opposite groups (reciprocal relaxation p. 167). Stretch your fingers, elbows, and arms upwards and backwards. It really will activate your whole body instead of allowing it to slump more and more as you work. Often if people thrust forward the pelvis when they are tired, the pelvis tips downwards and causes the low back to arch unduly and therefore to ache. Do pelvic tilt correction and control to alleviate this. Everything that I have said in this paragraph applies to dentists too. Now that they sit down to the job they may avoid varicose veins but they lean forward a lot and their spine can suffer accordingly.

Try to have shelves for instruments, bottles, brushes, towels, etc., and hooks for mirrors which you handle for every client, as high as may be comfortable for you to stretch to get what you want. In this way you again use the opposite arm muscles to those employed when dressing hair, or attending to teeth, and again you give these a little rest.

If your neck hurts you – and it often does – please don't stand and do head rolling on your seven unfortunate squashed neck joints. You will only damage them more. Do the three-point pull (p. 70). whenever you can and also stretch your back. After you have had lunch with your feet up, rest your head back against the chair, and then you can safely roll your supported head and bend it from side to side. Then tilt your head up to look at the ceiling. This will safely lubricate your neck joints and help them to carry your heavy head happily through the afternoon's work.

Lastly, I hope all hairdressers when washing hair, insist that the basin be behind the head so that the rim supports the nape of the neck. The pressure on the head when being rubbed can otherwise cause damage to the neck.

8. The over sixties

Anyone in this age group, as I am, will have found that they are caught in a nutcracker grip of fashion. Forty or more years ago, 'to be young was very heaven', was simply not true. The old were supposed to be 'wise and wonderful', our opinion was of no importance, and there seemed to be altogether too many of us. Now that we have entered the magic circle of the old, we haven't escaped from the nutcracker grip because fashion has swung round. Nowadays youth is the in thing. It is the new snobbery. There are still too many of our age group, and our opinions are still not asked.

I write this chapter to my contemporaries to say 'please come out of the nutcracker by yourself – by your own effort'. It can be done. Since you have survived for so long and through so many difficulties, you must have great resilience in your body and mind. Use that, to keep yourself healthy and happy, and above all part of the active community as long as you live. Remember that although Florence Nightingale spent the last fifty years of her life in bed, she was still working hard, reorganizing the nursing services of the army and in hospitals. Many young and middle-aged people are going to die long before we do. That is why we must regard ourselves as *living* people, not people about to 'pass on', 'pass over', or whatever phrase is favoured for dying.

The first thing is to preserve what you have got and to keep enjoying life, and being part of it. Of course I am speaking to those in normal health. Those who are in the care of their doctors will be acting on their advice. But even the old who are in delicate health can often help themselves enormously to recover.

WARMTH AND MOVEMENT

These go together. One of the strange things about getting older is that the temperature regulator in our low brain doesn't function very well. This means that older people get colder more easily, without being aware of it. If their temperature drops considerably they still may not feel cold, just weak and drowsy, and this is dangerous. It can make you really ill. So always see you are suitably clad for the weather.

Try never to sit for longer than half an hour. Get up and go and do something – anything – and so keep your circulation on the go. Sitting for a long time is so bad for muscles, joints, blood circulation, and general feelings. Remember too, your brain can't work properly without a good blood supply. Once you are allowed up after being ill, it is always better to put on a warm dressing-gown and slippers and go and do something. Don't sit about in a chair for a long time as this is very tiring; better to walk about and then lie down again.

Try the bed exercises in Chapter 7 and see if you like any of them. In any case do move about in bed and whenever you waken during the night, change your position. Remember 'movement is life' and you are still alive. Some oldish people lie in bed as though they were carved in marble. It seems a bit early to look like that. Your bed is just a resting place – not a tomb.

EXERCISE

This depends on what you are already able to do, and the object is to keep this going and perhaps increase some of it. In *Total fitness in 30 minutes a week* by Laurence E. Morehouse and Leonard Gross,[1] there are excellent suggestions for the simplest things that can be done. For example, when squeezing out the water from a face cloth, one should wring it, first one way and then the other, as firmly as possible. In this way two sets of muscles in the arms are strengthened. It does not matter how old or how disabled you may be, as long as the nerves are still attached to the muscles, they will work. Never give up.

You can arrange your own home to give you either daily exercise or ease in performance. It doesn't matter that you have always kept the coffee in that corner. Why not change it now? Put it on a higher shelf and you will have to stretch when you make a cup of coffee. So think out the placing of all the things you often use and decide whether you want to make it easier for yourself, or to give yourself a bit of exercise each time. You can have great fun doing all this. Decide whether you want to keep the potatoes under the sink which will give your back bending and raising exercise; or up on a shelf which gives stretching of your spine and upwards movements of your arms, at the same time strengthening your arm muscles and lubricating your shoulder and elbow joints. Or you could keep them outside in a shed, if you are lucky enough to have one, and if you walk briskly out to get them, in all weathers, you will exercise your legs and your lungs. Of course, if you need to conserve your strength, have everything possible within easy reach. Everyone should avoid straining the joints of the fingers and thumbs by lifting heavy bowls and casseroles. Try substituting lightweight polythene bowls and utensils wherever possible.

Apart from all these daily activities that I have suggested, you will be able to think up plenty more for yourself. If you want real exercises to do, read Chapters 5, 6, and 7, and select for yourself what you fancy. Certainly you shouldn't suddenly begin a hearty regime of exercises. Your aim should be to stop deterioration, and to keep all your joints gently oiled, and the muscles that open out and stretch your arms and legs comfortably strong. So often the dreaded 'middle-age spread' and 'bent old age' can be completely avoided by sensible diet and exercise. If in any doubt, consult your doctor.

WALKING

Do you 'pick up your feet' as you walk? So often older people stop using their ankle joints properly. Sometimes they tend to shorten their steps, and just push each foot in front of the other, practically flat on the ground. If you find you do this, first examine your shoes to see they really fit properly and don't wobble up and down as you walk. See that the heels are level – if they are not, take them to the cobbler, on your next walk. Try this: grasp a strong piece of furniture, or perhaps the kitchen sink, then rise up onto your toes and down again, as fast and as fully and as often as you can. Then walk quickly across the floor using your ankles as fully as possible. You will find it is much more satisfying than shuffling. Your forward foot should hit the floor heel down first with the toes up, then you put your weight onto that foot and lift the other behind you, which should also be bending at the ankle. When you bring the back foot forward, your knee should bend up in front before you lower the foot to the floor. Sometimes it helps to imagine you are stepping over something. Keep your head well up and swing your arms. The normal arm to swing forward is the one opposite the foot which is forward. So often I have had to help older people to relearn to walk properly, and they have always felt much better for it.

The slowing-down process begins so easily, and goes on so insidiously, and often people don't realize they are shuffling with their head down, and their arms close into their sides, instead of walking freely.

STICKS

If you have to use a stick for any reason, don't let it slow you down. It should help you to keep as fast a stride as possible. It is just there to support you, otherwise you should walk normally. If you are using a stick because you have something wrong with a leg, the stick is always carried in the hand opposite to the affected leg, never on the same side. If the stick is to help your balance and for general safety, use whichever hand suits you best. Don't bend down over it; press on the handle and stretch up away from it as you walk. Beware of too tall a stick, or you may damage your shoulder joint by the pressure. The greatest nuisance of a stick is that when you stop to do some job which needs both hands, it falls when you prop it against something. Try always to have a stick with a curved handle so you can hook it over your arm or in the front of your shirt, or any handy knob. Never put it on the roof of your car when you are getting in, or you may forget it and drive away – and that's another lost stick.

BREATHING

Every day try to hurry enough at some time so that you become breathless for a minute or so. Then your lungs are really given some extra work to do, and this keeps them active.

BALANCE

For as long as possible keep on standing up to put on socks, stockings, pants, and trousers. If necessary lean against the bed, so if you get wobbly you can fall onto it. Balancing on one leg is an excellent exercise, and the swaying as you get your socks or pants on, is marvellous activity for your back, tummy, leg, and foot muscles.

BATH

If you can't be bothered with the movements I have suggested in the bath exercises in Chapter 7, just wriggle about in any way you find easy and pleasant, and move your arms and legs likewise. Certainly get your legs stretched right out. Arch backwards and get your arms straight above your head; either do these movements all at once or in parts. We all tend to come forwards and inwards all our lives, so we should stretch out every day as often as possible. Do all movements gently and easily.

CHAIRS

There are some extraordinary chairs for the disabled nowadays, in which the seat helps to push you up, when you want to get up and out of them. This is splendid if you really need it, but often I have found that older people simply do not know how to get out of a chair using their own muscles properly, and so sit longer than is good for them, awaiting help to heave them out.

Your chair should have tall enough legs so that when you are sitting your knees are at a right angle and not bent up like a safety-pin. The back should be tall enough to put your head on it and it should have arms to lay your own arms along, when you are relaxing or having a cat nap.[2] Don't have a multitude of pillows so that you are wedged into the chair. Remember again 'movement is life' and you want to be able to move about inside your chair. In any case, I hope, as I have said, that you won't usually sit for longer than half an hour at a time.

GETTING UP

When you want to get up, if you are at all stiff or weak, try doing this. Stretch your arms above your head once or twice and arch your back while pressing your thighs down onto the seat, and turning your hips outwards. Straighten out your legs in front of you once or twice till you feel yourself more active and ready to get up. Then slide to the front of your chair, grasping the arms firmly, and put your feet forward on the floor, one slightly in front of the other. Now keep your head *up*, push *down* on your hands on the arms of the chair, and straighten up from your *hips*. You will then find yourself upright and in complete charge of yourself. Unfortunately people often drop their head and body forwards and struggle to get up after sitting motionless for hours. No wonder they find difficulty, and even fall. If you get your muscles ready to work and use your strongest muscles, i.e. your buttocks, you will find getting out of a chair not only easy but safe.

SITTING DOWN

Sitting down can also be a hazard if your muscles and joints are not as good as they once were, and you have got into bad habits. People are apt to approach the chair they intend to sit on, then, when they are about a yard away, they half turn their back towards it, bend forward, and aim their bottom at the seat. It is too easy to miss and fall. If they are lucky and their behind meets the seat, they positively collapse into the chair as though they had just completed some extraordinary muscular feat. This encourages the belief that they are frail and weak, when probably all they are is awkward.

To sit safely and easily is not difficult. Get that firmly in your head first. Walk straight up to the chair. When your legs are touching the front of the seat, turn around *completely upright*, until the backs of your legs are touching the same place. If you use a stick, hook it onto the side or back of the chair. Keep your head *up* facing forwards and working from your hips and knees, with a straight back, *slowly* lower yourself in a controlled manner, just steadying yourself with your hands on the arms of the chair, until you are on the seat of the chair. Do not thump yourself down.

It is often a good idea then, if you feel like it, to stand up again immediately in the proper manner and then sit once more, repeating once or twice to encourage yourself, and strengthen your muscles. I have often seen the gleam of self-pride and satisfaction come into old people's eyes, as they did this, and realized they weren't decrepit after all, and – what was more important to them – that they were still independent.

OUTINGS

Do try and get outside every day. Try to make these journeys interesting and exciting sometimes – not only just the dreary necessity to buy food. Use the great freedom of choice you have *because* you are over sixty – free of fashion, free of public opinion. You can do your own thing, but above all *do something*.

Alternative methods of movement

We have chosen several methods of exercise and movement to describe briefly. Addresses and books from which further details can be got are also listed. Of course there are many other kinds of exercise, dancing and physical training classes for the normal, the disabled and the athlete. We are mainly concerned with the average adult who wants to upgrade his physical health. We also hope the study of various ways of obtaining this will be of interest to all teachers of exercise. The wider any teacher's understanding of the subject, the better he or she will teach.

Aerobics

This is a system of exercise devised some years ago by Dr Kenneth H. Cooper of the United States Air Force Medical Corps. His latest findings are in *The New Aerobics* (Bantam paperback 1977, twenty-fourth printing). Aerobics refers to a variety of activities like walking, jogging and running for a measured time. These must be sufficiently far in distance and yet short in time to produce beneficial changes in the body, especially the action of the lungs, heart, and blood circulation. The idea is to increase the maximum amount of oxygen that the body can process in a given time, by exercise. You plan your own activity, working from charts compiled by Dr Cooper and his team from the evidence of thousands of people over several years. There is a 'starter program', then a twelve-minute test, which measures distance walked or run in twelve minutes. From this you judge your 'fitness category' according to your age and look out the programme suitable to your condition. All progressions are carefully arranged and throughout the book, precautions and advice are plentiful.

The charts are based on walking, running, cycling, swimming, handball, basketball and squash, but Dr Cooper approves of general body exercises for warm-up and cool-down periods. He says, 'Aerobics builds basic fitness and endurance. Calisthenics builds agility, co-ordination and muscular strength, particularly in the arms and upper torso. A highly conditioned person needs both.'

Total fitness in 30 minutes a week

This system has been composed by Dr Laurence E. Morehouse, Professor of Exercise Physiology and director of the Human Performance Laboratory at the University of California in Los Angeles. He has been working in this field for over forty years and was responsible, with others, for the studies of all kinds of body activity which enabled astronauts to work successfully on the Moon and return fit. He says, 'We wanted our money's worth.' The present programme is based on that experience.

Leonard Gross is a journalist who discovered how much teaching of exercise to lay people was out of date compared to the knowledge of the professional physiologists. So he teamed up with Professor Morehouse to write a book for the general public with up-to-date physiology and exercise information (*Total fitness in 30 minutes a week*, Granada 1977).

The Morehouse System is a personal approach to physical fitness including weight control, with a lavish amount of physiological explanation, precautions, and training in pulse taking. He is against all regimentation, competition, record breaking, over-development of muscle and heavy sweating. He reviews various popular systems and indicates what he thinks they lack. He maintains you need:

1. Muscle-building exercise
2. Muscle-endurance exercise to infuse it with blood capillaries
3. Circulo-respiratory development

This last is the most important and monitored all the time by your own pulse-taking. Exact instructions are given on how to do all this, and how to assess what is happening in your body from its own biofeedback system.

Great emphasis is placed on your own control of your training and progressive understanding of how to increase it. This is monitored by the person performing, using his own personal inclination and pulse rate as guides.

F/40 fitness on 40 minutes a week

This system was devised by a doctor and a gymnast who have specialized in, and written about, fitness for many years. The book is especially written for the unfit, not for the aspiring athlete. (*F/40: fitness on forty minutes a week*, by Malcolm Carruthers and Alistair Murray, Futura 1976.)

The first five short chapters explain clearly and simply why you should exercise, what happens during exercise, who needs it, when you should do it, when not, and finally how you begin and progress in the F40 system. Pulse-taking is described fully and is the basis of the control of the regime, which requires two or preferably three 15- to 20-minute sessions of activity each week. The exercises, which are clearly illustrated, are divided into mobility, strength, and light endurance for heart and lungs. There are three stages for each and then with added weights. The final chapter describes the medical data accumulated during trials of the system on middle-aged businessmen.

Jogging

Anyone in Britain who is taking up jogging should think about joining the National Jogging Club, 114 New Bond Street, London W1Y 9AB. He will receive a badge, advice on a healthy diet, information about recent and coming jogging events, joining a jogging club or starting a new one, and a most excellent handbook which is both scientific and sensible. This contains advice on clothing and shoes, how to warm up and how to warm down, how to jog and run, with a graded programme for beginners. It discusses in detail the physical and emotional effects of well-planned jogging. It gives the necessary precautions, and explains how to take the pulse easily without putting undue emphasis upon routine pulse-taking, or indeed any rigid routine. The writers, Leslie Kenton and Graham Jones, instead put great emphasis on each jogger getting to know the reactions of his own body, mental, physical and emotional. On this knowledge he is advised to plan and keep rearranging his own programme. Surely this is what exercise should be about.

Further reading: *The Complete Book of Running*, James Fixx, Chatto & Windus 1979.

Margaret Morris Movement

In the words of its brochure the 'Margaret Morris Movement is a unique system of exercise, movement and dance training which sets out to achieve a perfect balance between set exercises and free movement expression, and produces a complete harmony of body movement.' I was trained as a teacher in this method, as I mentioned in Chapter 1, and am therefore rather prejudiced in favour of it.

Margaret Morris Movement has three main divisions which are used in every class.

1. Greek 'Held' positions. There are six of these collected originally by Raymond Duncan (brother of Isadora Duncan) from Greek vases. They are static positions of the body held on bent hips, knees and ankles, and all involve balance and a twist at the waist, with varying static arm positions. They therefore amount to very strong static muscle work of the most important postural muscles, with particular control of the trunk rotators. This makes them very slimming for the abdominal bulge.

2. A mixed variety of exercises for stretching and strengthening all muscles, always performed to music, usually Schubert.

3. Improvisation of movements or dances often to improvised music or drum beats. All students are encouraged to compose dances, to design costumes, and to paint pictures.

There are ten standards of performance and four divisions; normal, remedial, athletic, aesthetic. In 1978 there were 138 registered teachers in Great Britain and Northern Ireland, and 53 in nine other countries. The number of attendances at classes in the year was 226,169. A resident summer school is held every year at a country house. Margaret Morris started her first school of movement in 1910. She died in February 1980 aged eighty-eight and took an active interest in all developments of her work until her death. All information can be obtained from the Administrator, Jim Hastie, at the International Association of MMM Ltd, Suite 3/4, 39 Hope Street, Glasgow G2 6AG.

The Women's League of Health and Beauty

The League was founded by Mrs Bagot-Stack in 1930. Although she is not now living, the League is still progressing under the supervision of her daughter and a council. There are 200 centres throughout England, Scotland and Wales and an overseas section. Classes are arranged in three grades: elementary, medium and advanced, all to music. There are also classes for movement with clubs, balls and hoops, and tap dancing. Classes are adapted for senior citizens, the disabled and children. There is a teachers' training course on a part-time basis over a three-year period. Public demonstrations are held, when the participants wear the League of Health and Beauty uniform of black pants and white blouse.

The Organising Secretary is Miss Peggy St Lo, Beaumont Cottage, Ditton Close, Thames Ditton, Surrey. Telephone 01-398-3719.

Mensendieck

Dr Bess Mensendieck became a household name throughout Europe in the 1930s and 1940s for her work on body health and beauty. Her early training was as a student of sculpture in Paris where she became more and more curious as to why some of the models had beautifully formed bodies while others had sags and bulges in all the wrong places. She decided to study medicine in order to find out. So started her life-long search into body mechanics and muscle function and the value of balanced posture and movement, which resulted in the Mensendieck System of Body Education. She set up many Mensendieck Institutes in Europe for teachers to be trained in her method. One of the teachers, Harriet Nyman, settled in London where she taught the Mensendieck Method. One of her pupils was Joanna Lewis who in turn became a teacher and taught Barbara Dale the Mensendieck System of Body Education.

There are classes based on Mensendieck at the Bodyworkshops, Lambton Squash Club, Lambton Place, Westbourne Grove, London W11 and The Hogarth Club, 1A Airedale Avenue, Chiswick W4. Classes in Yoga, relaxation and jazz exercises are also held.

Further reading:
Look Better, Feel Better, Bess Mensendieck, Harper & Row, New York 1954.
Fashion is Your Body: The Mensendieck–Nyman System of Exercises, Joanna Lewis and Molly Castle, Times Books 1974.

The Alexander Technique

The Alexander Technique is a form of teaching postural understanding and control initiated by F. Matthias Alexander at the end of the nineteenth century. He was an Australian who brought his method to London in 1904. Since then it has been widely taught in Britain, America and twelve other countries.

It is always taught on a one-to-one basis of teacher and pupil. The pupil is not taught exercises, but to recognize the 'Misuse of the Self' and to pause before performing any activity, such as standing up or sitting down, and then to direct how he performs this. The teacher helps by explanation and by passive movements with his hands, to further the perfect performance.

Alexander calls the 'Primary Control' the relationship between the head, neck and back in movement and on this foundation all postural training is made by very small adjustments of the muscular patterns that the pupil has already used. Alexander explains, 'You learn to inhibit and then direct your activity.' His mind – body technique emphasizes the recognition of the sensory stimuli of the body. It is said to lead to better health, greater body awareness, freedom to change, and the ability to choose or rid oneself of habits.

There are several centres whose addresses may be found in the local telephone book. Information may also be had from: The Society of Teachers of the Alexander Technique, 3 Albert Court, Kensington Gore, London SW7.

Further reading:
> *The Alexander Technique.* The essential writings of F. Matthias Alexander, selected and introduced by Edward Maisel, Thames & Hudson 1974.
> *The Alexander Principle – How to use your body*, Wilfred Barlow, Arrow Books 1975.
> *More Talk of Alexander*, edited by Wilfred Barlow, Gollancz 1978.
> *The Alexander Technique*, Sarah Barker, Bantam 1978.

Yoga

Yoga originated in India and its roots are as ancient as Sanskrit, the sacred language of India from which it takes its name. In Sanskrit, Yoga means union or yoke. It means linking yourself to a discipline through which you work towards balance and wholeness of body, mind and spirit.

Yoga is not only a physical discipline, as we often tend to think in the West today; it has many branches. For a full explanation of these and a good simple guide to the subject, please see Sophie Hoare's book *Yoga*. Practised fully, Yoga becomes a way of life, but we can choose what is useful for us and the physical postures are a very good start. Many Westerners find the relaxation and meditation aspects of Yoga very useful also.

Useful addresses:

Your local Adult Education Institute

British Wheel of Yoga, 445 High Road, Ilford, Essex IG1 1TR.

B. K. S. Iyengar Teachers' Association, 8 Vale Road, London N4. 1PZ.

Further reading:

Light On Yoga, B. K. S. Iyengar, Unwin Paperbacks 1971.

Yoga, Sophie Hoare, Macdonald Guidelines 1977.

Christian Yoga, Décharet, Search Press Ltd 1965.

The books of Dr Paul Brunton published by Rider & Co.

Tai-Chi Chuan, Karate, Judo

These are all forms of the martial arts which originated in China and Japan many centuries ago. They are still used widely in those countries as regimes for mind and body, and are increasingly popular in other countries too.

Tai-Chi Chuan consists in a variety of gentle continuous movements which require control of the whole body and demand concentration, co-ordination and poise. All movements are circular and develop balance and muscular control, rather than muscular bulk. It is based on the appreciation of opposites and contains much symbolism in its gestures.

Karate is a striking technique and Judo a grappling one. Judo has become very popular in the West today especially amongst young people, and has taken the place of boxing in many schools. It is an excellent form of exercise and can also be useful for self-defence. Judo is a very heavy exercise during which your pulse rate is likely to increase considerably and you sweat and breathe heavily. It works all parts of the body strongly, as you are moving yourself and another person who is also trying to move you. There are also a number of prearranged movement sequences, which you practise alone.

Information about the Chinese Arts and the instruction that is available throughout the world, can be obtained from The Chinese Cultural Arts Association, 90 Aldbanks, Dunstable, Bedfordshire.

Further reading:
The Chinese Art of Tai-Chi, Chee Soo, Gordon Cremonesi 1976.
Tai-Chi Chuan for Health and Beauty, Yang Ming-Shi, Bunka, Tokyo 1976.
Tai-Chi Chuan and I Ching, Da Lui, Routledge & Kegan Paul 1974.
Teach Yourself Judo, Syd Hoare, Hodder & Stoughton 1980.

References

CHAPTER 1 *pp.* 11–17

1 Gervis W. H., *Orthopaedics in General Practice*, Heinemann, 1958, pp. 46, 114.
2 *Physiotherapy Journal*, April 1977, pp. 120–123, Vasey and Crozier.
3 Cooper K. H., *The New Aerobics*, Bantam, 24th printing 1977, pp. 22–26, 122, 123, 154–169; Taylor, Eric, *Fitness After Forty*, John Murray, 1966, pp. 10–12, 140–155; *Living Well: The People Maintenance Manual*, ed. Tresidder, Mitchell Beazley, 1977, p. 120; Carruthers M. and Murray A., *F40: Fitness on Forty Minutes a Week*, Futura, 1978, chaps. 1–4, p. 33; Morgan R. E. and Adamson G. T., *Circuit Training*, G. Bell, 1961.
4 *Gray's Anatomy*, ed. Warwick and Williams, Longman, 35th edn 1973, pp. 800, 801; *Physiotherapy Journal*, December 1972, p. 404, J. Manning.
5 Quoted in Babsky, Khodorov, Kositsky, Zubkov, *Human Physiology*, MIR Moscow 1970, English translation 1975, pp. 148, 359.

CHAPTER 2 *pp.* 19–46

1 Collis, John Stewart, *Living with a Stranger*, Macdonald & Janes, 1978, p. 30.
2 Cooper J. M. and Glassow R. B., *Kinesiology*, Mosby, 4th edn 1976, pp. 16, 17.
3 Morehouse and Miller, *Physiology of Exercise*, Mosby, 7th edn 1976, pp. 256, 257; Cooper and Glassow, *Kinesiology*, pp. 25, 33, Bibliography pp. 336–346.
4 O'Connell and Gardner, *Understanding the Scientific Bases of Human Movement*, Williams & Wilkins, 1st edn 1972, pp. 85, 86.
5 Mensendieck B. M., *Look Better, Feel Better*, Harper & Row, 1954, p. 38.
6 Sinclair, David, *Human Growth after Birth*, Oxford University Press, 2nd edn 1973, p. 33.
7 Lockhart R. D., *Living Anatomy*, Faber, 5th edn 1959, p. 72.
8 *Report of the Task Group on Reference Man*, ICRP, Pergamon, 1975, p. 43.
9 Moorehead, Alan, *The White Nile*, Penguin, new edn 1973.
10 *Human Growth after Birth*, pp. 105, 115.
11 Raeburn J. K. and H. A., *Anatomy, Physiology and Hygiene*, John Murray, 4th edn 1975, p. 60.
12 Pappus, Alexandr., *Collectis* Book VIII, Proposition 10. Pliny the Elder, *Natural History* Book VII.

13 Cooper and Glassow, *Kinesiology*, pp. 37–49.
14 *Understanding the Scientific Bases of Human Movement*, p. 47.
15 Gardiner, Dena M., *The Principles of Exercise Therapy*, G. Bell, 3rd edn 1973, p. 12; *Understanding the Scientific Bases of Human Movement*, p. 43; Thompson, Clem W., *Manual of Structural Kinesiology*, Mosby, 8th edn 1977, pp. 127, 133.
16 Taylor, Eric, *Strength and Stamina Training*: A Guide to Training with Weights, Circuit Training and Isometric exercises, John Murray, 1970.
17 Wells, Katharine, *Kinesiology*, Saunders, 5th edn 1971, pp. 83–89, Newton's Laws; *The Principles of Exercise Therapy*, pp. 10–14.
18 Karpovich P. V. and Sinning W. E., *Physiology of Muscular Activity*, Saunders, 1971, p. 45; Rasch P. J. and Burke R. K., *Kinesiology and Applied Anatomy*, Lea & Febiger, 6th edn 1978, pp. 127–141.
19 Cooper and Glassow, *Kinesiology*, pp. 57, 58.
20 Basmajian J. V., *Primary Anatomy*, Williams & Wilkins, 7th edn 1976, pp. 120, 121.
21 Guyton A. C., *Function of the Human Body*, Saunders, 4th edn 1974, pp. 242–250; Grollman S., *The Human Body. Its Structure and Physiology*, Macmillan USA, 4th edn 1978, pp. 170–174; Mackean, Don and Jones, Brian, *Introduction to Human and Social Biology*, John Murray, 3rd edn 1977, p. 147.
22 Mitchell, Laura, *Simple Relaxation*, John Murray 1977, pp. 37, 38.
23 *Manual of Structural Kinesiology*, pp. 46, 47.
24 *The Human Body. Its Structure and Physiology*, pp. 161, 162; Basmajian J. V., *Muscles Alive* (Electromyography), Williams & Wilkins, 2nd edn 1967, pp. 86–88.
25 *Function of the Human Body*, p. 251; Thomas, Vaughan, *Exercise Physiology*, Crosby Lockwood Staples 1975, pp. 36, 37.
26 Wells, *Kinesiology*, pp. 175, 176, 402, 403.
27 *Primary Anatomy*, pp. 315–320; Last R. J., *Anatomy Regional and Applied*, Churchill Livingstone, 6th edn 1978, pp. 536–540; Wells, *Kinesiology*, chap. 11; *Gray's Anatomy*, pp. 798–825 (especially joints pp. 800–804); *Simple Relaxation*, p. 23.
28 Wells, *Kinesiology*, pp. 172–174.
29 *Primary Anatomy*, p. 119.
30 Guyton A. C., *Structure and Function of the Nervous System*, Saunders, 1972, pp. 158–168.
31 Beevor C., *The Croomian Lectures on muscular movements*, delivered at Royal College of Physicians, London 1903, Macmillan.
32 *Function of the Human Body*, pp. 325–327; *Structure and Function of the Nervous System*, p. 201.
33 *Exercise Physiology*, p. 328.
34 Cooper and Glassow, *Kinesiology*, p. 67.

35 Sherrington, *The Integrative Action of the Nervous System*, Murray Printing Co., Forge Village, Mass., 2nd edn 1947, Foreword, p. xiii.

36 *Introduction to Human and Social Biology*, pp. 28, 89, 98.

37 *The New Aerobics*, Bantam, pp. 15–19, 169.

38 *The Human Body. Its Structure and Physiology*, pp. 112–115.

39 *The New Aerobics*, pp. 166, 168; *Introduction to Human and Social Biology*, p. 28.

40 *Physiology of Exercise*, p. 166.

41 *Simple Relaxation*, pp. 25–28.

42 *Human Growth After Birth*, p. 31.

43 a. Morehouse and Gross, *Total Fitness in Thirty Minutes a Week*, Mayflower, 1977, pp. 182–188.

    b. *Introduction to Human and Social Biology*, pp. 32–39.

    c. *Function of the Human Body*, pp. 327–330; *The New Aerobics*, p. 166; *Total Fitness in Thirty Minutes a Week*, pp. 21–25.

    d. Mackean D. G., *Introduction to Biology*, John Murray, 1977, pp. 137–143.

    e. *Function of the Human Body*, pp. 322–324.

    f. *Structure and Function of the Nervous System*, pp. 71, 81, 82, 200, 201.

    g. *Physiology of Muscular Activity*, pp. 99, 100, chaps. 15, 16.

    h. *Structure and Function of the Nervous System*, pp. 241, 242.

    i. *The New Aerobics*, pp. 15–17.

    k. Cooper and Glassow, *Kinesiology*, pp. 64, 66.

    l. *Simple Relaxation*, p. 14.

    m. *The New Aerobics*, pp. 23–26, 29, 43, 167; *F40: Fitness on Forty Minutes a Week*, pp. 30, 31.

CHAPTER 3 *pp.* 47–65

1 Anderson J., *Grant's Atlas of Anatomy*, Williams & Wilkins, 7th edn 1978, colour illustrations; *Anatomy Regional and Applied*, pp. 243–245, 255–259; the *Manual of Structural Kinesiology* has all the muscles of the body illustrated separately and in colour.

2 Bourne, Gordon, *Pregnancy*, Cassell 1972, pp. 229, 230.

3 Cunningham D. J., *Manual of Practical Anatomy*, ed. Romanes, Vol. 2 'Thorax and abdomen', Oxford University Press, 14th edn 1977, pp. 134, 135, 149.

4 *Grant's Atlas of Anatomy*, Section 2, pp. 120, 121b.

5 *Grant's Atlas of Anatomy*, Section 1, p. 46; *Anatomy Regional and Applied*, p. 217.

6 *Gray's Anatomy*, pp. 517, 518, 719, 1316, 1317; *Grant's Atlas of Anatomy* Section 1, illustrations 46, 47, 50, 51, 53, 61, 62, 82–84. Section 2, illustrations 26, 36a, 49, 120, 121a, 121b, 350. Section 3, illustrations 10, 11, 39, 63, 64.

7 Barlow W., *More Talk of Alexander*, Gollancz 1978, p. 115.

8 *Grant's Atlas of Anatomy*, Section 3, illustrations 12–15, 21, 67, 73; *Anatomy Regional and Applied*, pp. 323–327; Mandelstam D., *Incontinence*, Heinemann 1977, pp. 6–8, 21, 22; *Physiotherapy Journal*, August 1978, p. 236 D. Mandelstam.

9 *Primary Anatomy*, pp. 138–141.

10 *Grant's Atlas of Anatomy*, Section 2, illustrations 5–9, 11, 12, 119, 120, 122–124; *Manual of Practical Anatomy*, pp. 78, 81, 82; Daniels L. and Worthingham C., *Muscle Testing*, Saunders, 3rd edn 1972, pp. 22–24; *Anatomy Regional and Applied*, pp. 255–259; Wells, *Kinesiology*, pp. 338–342, 361–362.

11 *Primary Anatomy*, pp. 30, 31.

12 Wells, *Kinesiology*, pp. 332–337; *Muscle Testing*, pp. 24–26; *Grant's Atlas of Anatomy*, Section 5, illustrations 25–29, 31, Section 6, illustration 30; *Primary Anatomy*, p. 143.

13 *Grant's Atlas of Anatomy*, Section 2, illustration 10; *Manual of Practical Anatomy*, pp. 78, 81, 82.

14 *Fitness After Forty*, p. 54; *Physiotherapy Journal*, December 1975, p. 383, letter J. A. Carron Brown FRCOG; Noble, Elizabeth, *Essential Exercises for the Childbearing Year*, John Murray 1978, pp. 16–18, 64; *Manual of Structural Kinesiology*, p. 53; Wells, *Kinesiology*, p. 398.

CHAPTER 4 *pp.* 66–80

1 *Reader's Digest*, July 1978, p. 151.

2 Anthony and Kolthoff, *Textbook of Anatomy and Physiology*, Mosby USA, 9th edn 1975, p. 125.

3 *Human Growth after Birth*, pp. 95, 105, 113–117.

4 Cooper and Glassow, *Kinesiology*, p. 193; *Human Physiology*, pp. 159–164.

5 *Primary Anatomy*, p. 172.

6 Basmajian J. V., *Grant's Method of Anatomy*, Williams & Wilkins, 9th edn 1975, p. 352.

7 Cooper and Glassow, *Kinesiology*, p. 192; *Muscles Alive*, pp. 149–153.

8 *Primary Anatomy*, p. 172.

9 *Introduction to Human and Social Biology*, p. 122 fig. 16.30.

10 *Gray's Anatomy*, pp. 583, 585.

11 Wells, *Kinesiology*, chap. 20.

12 *The Human Body. Its Structure and Physiology*, p. 370.

13 *Exercise Physiology*, pp. 68–70, 117, 118.

14 *Function of the Human Body*, p. 215.

15 *Grant's Method of Anatomy*, p. 418; *Anatomy Regional and Applied*, p. 218, 222; Gaskell B. V. and Webber B. A., *The Brompton Hospital Guide to Chest Physiotherapy*, Blackwell, 2nd edn 1973, pp. 1–4.

16 *Gray's Anatomy*, p. 519; *Simple Relaxation*, illustration p. 95.

17 *Grant's Method of Anatomy*, p. 418.

18 *Textbook of Anatomy and Physiology*, p. 300; Nilsson, Lennart, *Behold man*, Harrap 1974, pp. 81–93.

19 *The Human Body. Its Structure and Physiology*, pp. 269, 276.

20 Shephard, Roy, *The Fit Athlete*, Oxford University Press 1978, pp. 90–93.

21 *The Brompton Hospital Guide to Chest Physiotherapy*, pp. 2–3.

22 *The Human Body. Its Structure and Physiology*, pp. 349–352.

23 *Function of the Human Body*, chap. 18; *The Human Body. Its Structure and Physiology*, pp. 349–361; *Anatomy Regional and Applied*, pp. 212–220; *Primary Anatomy*, pp. 46–48, 136, 137, 141, 142, figures 235, 236, 377, 424, 427.

24 *The Human Body. Its Structure and Physiology*, p. 361.

25 Lum, Dr L. C., *Breathing Exercises in the Treatment of Hyperventilation and Chronic Anxiety States*, Papworth Hospital.

26 *Anatomy Regional and Applied*, p. 220; *The Brompton Hospital Guide to Chest Physiotherapy*, pp. 1–4; *Simple Relaxation*, pp. 92–97.

27 *The New Aerobics*, p. 46; *The Fit Athlete*, pp. 90–93; *Textbook of Anatomy and Physiology*, pp. 301–303, 308–314.

28. *Human and Social Biology*, Chap. 11.

29 *Function of the Human Body*, pp. 28–29.

CHAPTER 8 *pp.* 196–201

1 *Total Fitness in 30 Minutes a Week*, pp. 139–141; Shepard R., *Physical Activity and Aging*, Croom Helm 1978, pp. 85, 102–106, 147–149, 154; *The Fit Athlete*, p. 91.

2 *Simple Relaxation*, pp. 45, 46, 54.

Further reading

'Arts in Therapy, The', *Physiotherapy Journal*, 10 March 1978.

Black, Stephen, *Mind and Body*, Kimber, 1969.

Bourne, Geoffrey (ed.), *Structure and Function of Muscle*, Academic Press, 2nd edn 1973, Vol. III.

Braithwaite M., *Medau Rhythmic Movement*, The Medau Society of Great Britain, 3rd edn 1976.

Broer, Marion R., *Efficiency of Human Movement*, Saunders, 3rd edn 1973.

Broer, Marion R., *An Introduction to Kinesiology*, Prentice-Hall, 1968.

Bryant, John, *Jogging*, Hamlyn, 1979.

Carrier and Shibata (ed.), *Factors Influencing Vascular Reactivity*, Igaku Shoin, Tokyo and New York, 1977.

Chaplin, Mary, *Gardening for the Physically Handicapped and Elderly*, Batsford, in association with the Royal Horticultural Society, 1978.

Costonis M. N. (ed.), *Therapy in Motion*, University of Illinois Press, 1978.

Cratty, Bryant J., *Movement Behaviour and Motor Learning*, Lea & Febinger, 3rd edn 1974.

Davis A. M., *Feeling Great*, The Health Education Council, London, and The Scottish Health Education Unit, Edinburgh, n.d.

Dineen, Jacqueline, *Rewarding Retirement*, Thorsons, 1978.

Directory for the Disabled, Woodhead-Faulkner, 1979.

Gillie, Oliver (ed.), *The Sunday Times Book of Body Maintenance*, Michael Joseph, 1977.

Gore, Irene, *Age and Vitality*, Allen & Unwin, 1973.

Grandjean E., *Fitting the Task to the Man: an Ergonomic Approach*, Taylor & Francis, 1969.

Grant R. (ed.), *Nobel Symposium: Muscular Afferents and Motor Control*, John Wiley, 1966.

Green J. H., *Basic Clinical Physiology*, Oxford University Press, 3rd edn 1978.

Guttmann, Sir Ludwig, *Sport for the Physically Handicpped*, UNESCO, 1976 (available free of charge from the Secretariat, UNESCO, 7 Place de Fontenoy, 75700 Paris, France).

Hamilton W. J. (ed.), *Textbook of Human Anatomy*, Macmillan, 2nd edn 1976.

Healey, Colin, *Methods of Fitness*, Kaye & Ward, 1973.

Kennedy, Pat, *The Moving Body*, Faber, 1979.

Knuttgen H. G. (ed.), *Neuromuscular Mechanisms for Therapeutic and Conditioning Exercise*, University Park Press, 1977.

Lum L. C., 'Hyperventilation: the Tip and the Iceberg', *Journal of Psychosomatic Research*, Vol. 19, pp. 375–383, Pergamon Press, 1975.

McConnaill, M.A. and Basmajian, J. V., *Muscles and Movements*, Williams and Wilkins, 2nd edn 1978.

Man's Body, Corgi, 1977.

Miller, Jonathan, *The Body in Question*, Cape, 1978.

Murray, Jan, *Dance Now*, Penguin, 1979.

Nourse A. E., *The Body*, Life Books, Pocket edn 1969, pp. 150–151.

Rasch P. J. and Burke R. K., *Kinesiology and Applied Anatomy: Science of Human Movement*, Lea & Febinger, 5th edn 1974.

Samuels, Michael and Bennett, Harold Zina, *The Well Body Book*, Wildwood House, 1974.

Smith, Anthony, *The Body*, Allen & Unwin, 2nd edn 1970.

Spence, Dale W., *Essentials of Kinesiology*, Lea & Febinger, 1975.

Stinson, David and Lough, Richard, *Aquatics Recreation and Fitness in Water*, Harper, 1973.

Taylor, Gordon Rattray, *The Natural History of the Mind*, Secker & Warburg, 1979.

Index

Also from John Murray

SIMPLE RELAXATION
THE PHYSIOLOGICAL METHOD
FOR EASING TENSION

LAURA MITCHELL

'Most useful for learning a good technique for relaxation quickly. The explanations are clear and directions simple to follow, the chapters on practical application of the method in everyday situations excellent.'—*Mother and Baby*

'This excellent book fulfils the purpose for which it was written – to help people who find themselves tense and tired and unable to relax. No extravagant claims are made but sound reasons are propounded for the techniques advocated, based on currently accepted physiological principles. The writing is attractive, informal and conversational in style without being arch. Clear diagrams and photographs complement the text admirably.'—*Nursing Times*

'Her method of relaxation is pleasantly easy – no meditation, or complicated exercises – and her section for antenatal, labouring and postnatal mothers should be particularly helpful'—*British Medical Journal*

'A practical book for the layman which all professional people dealing with stress and tension in others should read. Health, life style and relationships can only improve by the use of this method'—*Physiotherapy*

126 pp (paperback)
drawings and diagrams throughout